A Family Doctor's Guide to

UNDERSTANDING

AND

PREVENTING CANCER

ENVIRONMENTAL RISKS AND SOLUTIONS

S.R. KAURA, M.D.

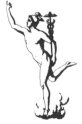

HEALTHPRESS

P.O. DRAWER 1388
SANTA FE, NM 87504

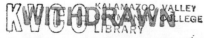

Published 1991 by Health Press
P.O. Drawer 1388
Santa Fe NM 87504

Library of Congress Cataloging-in-Publication Data

Kaura, S. R., 1948-
    A Family Doctor's Guide to Understanding
          and Preventing Cancer / S.R. Kaura
      p. cm.
  ISBN 0-929173-03-1 $24.95
  1. Cancer--Popular Works. 2. Cancer--Prevention. 3. Cancer--Etiology.
  I. Title.

RC263.K278 1989
616'.99'4--dc20   89-26893
                                   CIP

In memory of my dear uncle, the late Professor Ram Gopal Kaura, Ph.D., who devoted his life to educating society.

Nothing in life is to be feared:
It is only to be understood.

Marie Curie

NOTE

The information presented in this book has been obtained from authentic and reliable sources. Reprinted material has been printed with permission from the sources given. References are listed in bibliographies at the end of each chapter. Although great care has been taken to ensure the accuracy of the information presented, the author and the publisher cannot assume responsibility for the validity of all the materials or the consequences for their use.

Acknowledgments

I am very much indebted to the professional assistance by Health Press, especially Kathleen Schwartz for showing great sensitivity, guidance and overall direction to this project. My special thanks to Kriszti Fehérváry for her skillful editing. Assisting in the research for this book were P. Salamone, Lisa Alfano, Mary Beth Victor; my secretaries; Diane O'Keefe of Wyandotte Hospital Library, and other librarians at the University of Michigan and Receiving Hospital. Typing was done by Cyndi Hoops. Sample menus were prepared by Mary Hillcoat. Editorial assistance was provided by Ann Rousch and Marge des Lauriers. Special thanks to Drs. A. Prasad, V. Sanghi and P. Khan for reviewing the manuscript. I would like to acknowledge a special thanks to Carl Just and Susan Peterson of Wyandotte Hospital for their support. Due to constraints of space, many names have not been mentioned; this does not lessen the importance of their contributions. Last, but not least, my love and appreciation to my family for their support, inspiration and understanding — without which this book could never have been possible.

I apologize in advance for the inevitable errors which will be discovered in a manuscript of this magnitude. I would welcome any suggestions or comments regarding this edition for use in future editions.

S. R. Kaura, M.D.

...a challenging undertaking by Dr. S.R. Kaura...a good job of putting together the pertinent information for practicing physicians and lay public.

Ananda S. Prasad, M.D., Ph.D.
Professor of Medicine and
   Director of Research
Wayne State University School of Medicine
Detroit, Michigan

CONTENTS

Preface

Cancer is a horrifying group of almost 200 different diseases, more than 90 percent of which are related to environmental causes. Cancer threatens a large segment of the population, and incidence is increasing at the rate of approximately one percent annually. The cure rates run at only 50 percent, so many patients die within five years of the diagnosis. All these statistics show that with our present strategy focusing on treatment, we are losing the war against cancer. In modern medicine, prevention of diseases is quite a success story, whether it is in terms of heart disease or infectious diseases. Similarly for cancer, prevention is a very practical and promising, but often neglected solution. Prevention can be achieved by controlling the cancer causing agents around us. Here, we as individuals have to take responsibility and become involved in taking steps to reduce our risk of getting cancer.

My initial interest in this topic came from my clinical experiences with my patients over the last ten years. As I was getting more involved in doing the related research on this topic and attending cancer prevention seminars, I found no book on the market that would comprehensively cover the subject of cancer as an environmental disease which could be prevented.

I was astonished to discover a great deal of confusion and misunderstanding on the subject in talking to patients, colleagues, friends and family. "Everything causes cancer," they worried, "how can you prevent it?" Believe me, we would be in a lot of trouble if this were true. Fortunately, only a small number of things cause cancer. We can all take a number of measures on a personal level to reduce our risks.

Addictions like tobacco, marijuana, alcohol, intravenous drug abuse and steroids are well known causes of cancer. We can all take steps in educating our family and friends who are addicted, in seeking help through rehabilitation programs to get rid of these addictions.

Eating a well balanced diet, low in fat and cholesterol and high in fiber, is "killing both birds (cancer and heart disease) with one stone." By maintaining a near ideal body weight with diet and exercise, we can virtually walk away from cancer. Vitamins and minerals are scoring very high on the cancer prevention and treatment front.

In growing food, both nationally and internationally, the indiscriminate and careless use of dangerous pesticides and fertilizers is leaving dangerous residues on our food. There is a real need for placing severe restrictions on the manufacture, sale and use of pesticides.

A promiscuous love life is a glamorous thing only on soap operas and in movies. In real life it can lead to cancer and AIDS. Many sexually transmitted diseases, especially viral, lead to cancer. The most important diseases in this category are HIV infection leading to AIDS, Hepatitis B infection leading to liver cancer, and Human Papilloma Virus causing genital warts and cancer. Many vaccines are being developed against these sexually transmitted viruses and cancer, but the competence of the immune system as the defense system of our body is critical. Miracles of nature, where the immune system wipes out well established cancers, are well known. Good emotional health and good nutrition are key factors for a strong immune system.

We are exposed to many items in our personal hygiene that contain carcinogenic ingredients, such as synthetic hair dye, talcum powder, nail polishes, blushes, and certain hair shampoos.

We play with cancer causing agents through some of our hobbies, especially handling dyed maggots in fishing, ceramics, painting, gardening or changing oil in the car. Even housework can be a cancer hazard, which is not such good news for housewives. Pantries of some homes look like chemical labs.

In seeking medical care, there are dangers to both the medical professionals and the patients. Chemotherapy and radiation treatments for cancer patients and anti-rejection drugs given to transplant patients act like double-edged swords, treating our ailments now but leaving us at a higher risk for second cancer later in life.

Work place exposure to carcinogenic agents is a major contributor to the cancer problem. Asbestos, pesticides, benzene, and related solvents, permanent dyes, formaldehyde and chlorinated solvents are a few examples. Much more can be done to reduce work place exposure.

The air we breathe is getting more polluted—both at work and at home. Airtight buildings, which bottle up pollutants, are making the people who work in them sick. At home, cigarette smoke, cooking and heating appliances, construction material and radon are taking their toll on us. The water we drink is becoming polluted because of toxic dumps, improper sewage disposal, industrial discharges and leaking land-fills. A large part of this problem can be solved by recycling and proper disposal of household garbage. The pollutants in the air, water and in the soil are ending up in our food supply and eventually into our bodies. What a price for civilization!

In a small percentage of cancers, heredity or family history puts us at a higher risk of getting cancer. As researchers better understand genetics, we will be better able to control hereditary risk—and perhaps even change the genes responsible for passing cancer from generation to generation.

Early detection of cancer can be achieved in many ways: by assessing our personal risk with self-questionnaires, learning the proper techniques of self-examination, and being part of screening programs. Finally, we can follow a recommended schedule for cancer related checkups from our family physician.

This book is designed to make the complex topic of cancer prevention easy to understand. I have used simple, straightforward language, many illustrations and a touch of humor with appropriate cartoons. If all the counsel given in this book is carefully followed, I believe in the next few decades hundreds and thousands of lives could be saved, as well as billions of dollars in health care costs. With today's scarcity of resources and cost-conscious society, we don't have any choice but to go all out in our efforts to prevent cancer.

S.R. Kaura, M.D.

Introduction

WINNING THE WAR AGAINST CANCER

Cancer is a word that disturbs us. It carries an image of a deadly invader; it is chilling because it can mean a death sentence. Yet, in many cases cancer is treatable and frequently preventable.

Cancer, the second most common cause of death in the United States, can be found in many forms of life, including plants, animals, insects, and human beings. Affecting every age group and knowing no geographic boundaries, cancer is a public health problem facing all of us.

Drs. Michael Bunk and Richard S. Rivlin of Memorial Sloan Kettering Cancer Center estimate that by the year 2000, roughly 40 percent of the human population will be attacked by some form of cancer, and may cause 25 percent of all deaths.[1] If these projections hold true, cancer will be the number' one cause of death in the next century. As other causes of death such as heart disease and infections decline and more people live to ripe old ages, death rates from cancer continue to rise. According to the World Health Organization there were a total of 5.8 million cases of cancer worldwide and 4.3 million deaths in 1984: 2.3 million deaths were in developing countries where 75 percent of the world's population lives, and two million in the industrialized world where the remaining 25 percent lives.

One million people in the United States are afflicted by some form of cancer each year. According to the American Cancer Society, 462,000 people died of cancer in 1985 alone—accounting for approximately 18 percent of all deaths that year.[2] Although these numbers are constantly on the rise, in many cases cancer could be prevented.

Cancer is expensive, not only in terms of human life, but also in terms of medical care costs. The overall medical costs of cancer in the United States, according to a study done by the National Center of Health Statistics, was 71 billion dollars for the year 1985—roughly 10 percent of the total health care budget. Out of this amount, the American Cancer Society found that 21.8 billion went to direct costs, 8.6 billion to lost productivity, and 41.2 billion for indirect costs.[3]

Present Strategies for Early Detection and Treatment

We are dealing with the problem of cancer currently by focusing primarily on research and treatment. Rates of success of different cancer treatments vary, according to a study by the General Accounting Office.[4] There have been important gains in the treatment of less common cancers like lymphatic cancers, leukemias and testicular cancer. Some gains have been made in the treatment of bladder and prostate cancers. Small gains have been made in the treatment of most of the common cancers like breast, lung, colon, cervix and uterus, and head and neck cancers. Practically no gains have been made in the treatment of stomach cancer. A more important gain is the significant improvement in the quality of life of many cancer patients. One half of these patients are living five years or longer after treatment of the initial cancer.

There has been a significant effort on the part of the American Cancer Society to educate the public about cancer illnesses associated with smoking, sunlight exposure and diet, and also about early detection through the use of pap smears, breast exams, and the like. However, the overall thrust of efforts against cancer are directed at early detection and treatment and less at primary prevention, despite the fact that many cancers can be prevented. The results of this strategy are disappointing.

Are we really winning the war against cancer? The answer must be "no", in spite of the statistics mentioned above. Dr. John Bailar III of the Harvard School of Public Health and Dr. Elaine Smith of the University of Iowa, dealt with this question directly. They concluded that the incidence of cancer is rising at one percent annually while the cancer death rate rises at the same rate, in spite of the money being poured into research and treatment of cancer.[5] These doctors believe that we need to re-evaluate our strategies in the war against cancer. The intensive efforts which have focussed primarily on treatment over the past 35 years appear to have failed.

There is a vast body of research that suggests more than 90 percent of cancers are environmental in origin, says John Higginson, a senior investigator at the Universities Associated for Research and Education in Pathology in Maryland.[6] By "environmental" I mean those things our bodies are exposed to through the air we breathe, the food we eat and water we drink, the places we work. Our exposure to infectious diseases is also considered an environmental factor.

Our experience with environmental diseases has shown that by controlling risk factors we can bring down mortality rates. An example is heart disease caused by high cholesterol and hypertension; because of educational campaigning by the American Heart Association, mortality rates from heart disease were reduced by 25 percent. Similarly, we have done well in the area of infectious diseases such as small pox and polio, and tremendous progress is also being made in research on AIDS.

There are various environmental causes for cancer. No one is sure of the exact percentages of cancers caused by specific agents, but according to the best figures available, the consensus is as follows: smoking and other tobacco use is responsible for about 35 percent of all cancers, radiation for five percent, diet for 35 percent, viruses for about five percent, heredity for five to ten percent,[7] and industrial chemicals for 30 to 40 percent. Dr. Samuel Epstein of the University of Illinois thinks that all of these factors may be controllable.[8]

"Love is fine, but it takes money to buy wine," says the proverb; the same is true about the necessity of adequate funding for cancer prevention. Out of a total yearly budget of the one billion dollars allocated to the National Cancer Institute, less than one percent is earmarked for prevention, according to Dr. Neil Barnard of George Washington University. Considering the magnitude of the cancer problem, this amount is minimal. Barnard feels we could save 500 million dollars in treatment costs if only the incidence of breast cancer were reduced by ten percent through a lowfat diet.[9] One can imagine the savings if principles of prevention were applied to all cancers.

Prevention Works

Many public health experts feel prevention is the key to winning the war against the cancer epidemic. Drs. Bailar and Smith feel that we should take the prevention route to realize great savings in both lives and dollars. As a family doctor, I know how difficult it is to treat established conditions. For every physician, prevention is the best tool. According to conservative American Cancer Society estimates, 164 thousand lives could be saved annually if cancer prevention and detection techniques were fully implemented.[10]

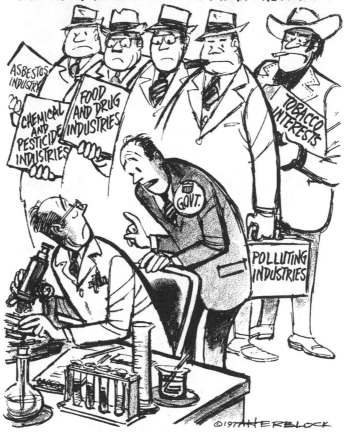

Reprinted with permission by Herblock on All Fronts. *New American Library, 1980*

In the next chapter we will deal will the issues of why and how cancer can be prevented. Research scientists have confirmed what we clinicians have known for centuries, that an ounce of prevention is worth a pound of cure.

BIBLIOGRAPHY NOTES

1. Michael Bunk and Richard S. Rivlin, *Current Concepts and Perspectives in Nutrition,* (March 1987)

2. American Cancer Society, *Cancer Facts and Figures*, (1987)

3. *Ibid.*

4. General Accounting Office, *Journal of the American Medical Association*, (May 22, 1987)

5. J. Bailar, and E. Smith, "Progress Against Cancer," *New England Journal of Medicine*, (May 8, 1986)

6. John Higginson, *Hospital Practice.* November, 1983

7. Jerome Mormorstein, "Packaging Cancer Prevention Via the Doctor," *Medical Tribune*, (March 26, 1986) and (April 3, 1985)

8. Samuel Epstein, and J. Swartz, "The Fallacies of Lifestyle Cancer Theories," *Nature*, (Jan. 15, 1981)

9. Neil Barnard, "Prevention Must Take Priority," *Medical World News*, (June 27, 1988)

10. American Cancer Society. op.cit.

CHAPTER ONE

CANCER: ENVIRONMENTAL AND PREVENTABLE

Cancer has been recognized as a disease for centuries. Tumors have been discovered in Egyptian mummies and references were made to cancer in ancient Egyptian writings as long ago as 1500 B.C. Even dinosaur fossils show evidence of cancer. Hippocrates, the father of medicine, gave the disease the name "cancer" (Greek for crab) because it spread through tissues like the movements of a crab.

The thinking that in many cases cancer may be caused by environmental factors has evolved over the past two centuries. An historical account of the research on this theory provides clues.

Chemicals were the first to be suspected as a *cause* of cancer. In 1775 an English physician, Percival Pott, found that chimney sweepers suffered from scrotal cancer because of extended exposure to the hot soot in chimneys. In 1895 Dr. L. Rehn, a physician in Germany, found bladder cancer in three workers involved in production of Aniline dyes. Later, experiments done on animals with dyes resulted in bladder cancer. In 1915 two Japanese scientists, Dr. K. Yamagiwa and Dr. K. Ichikawa of the University of Tokyo, applied coal tar to rabbits' ears and produced skin cancer.[1] By the early part of the 20th century the theory that chemicals were the cause of many of our cancers was well established.

Paul Unna suspected sunlight as the cause of skin cancer as early as 1894. He noticed a higher incidence of skin cancer among people who developed a sailor's weathered skin from excessive exposure to sunshine for prolonged periods of time. G. M. Findlay showed in 1928 that ultraviolet light could cause cancer in mice.[2] Finally, in 1941, H.P. Rusch and his associates found that the ultraviolet portion of sunlight caused skin cancer in human beings.[3]

A few years after the discovery of X rays in 1895 by a German doctor named Roentgen, it was found that the doctors and technicians who used X ray machines developed skin cancer on skin areas exposed to the rays. Although radium and other radioactive materials were discovered in 1898, it was not until 1945, after the Second World War, that people realized the horrifying effects of radiation. The Japanese exposed to radiation from the two atomic bombs developed almost every kind of cancer known.

Radon gas had been suspected as a cause of lung cancer in miners in the early 1900s. We have discovered more recently that radon gas—which has been found to be carcinogenic—leaks into our homes from underground deposits of radioactive materials.

In the later half of the 19th century different microbes were found to cause bacterial diseases. At the same time, suspicion was growing that some cancers could be caused by bacterial and viral infection. The first experiment in this new field was conducted in 1911 by Peyton Rous, a research scientist in the Rockefeller Foundation in New York.[4] He was able to pass on a cancer from one chicken to another. Later, there were many experiments in which cancer-causing viruses were passed from one laboratory animal to another. We are aware today of a number of viruses that cause cancer in human beings: hepatitis B causes liver cancer, and Human Papilloma Virus causes genital cancers in males and females.

Hormones were first discovered to have a relationship to cancer in 1916 by Drs. Lathrop and Loeb, who demonstrated that the castration of female mice prevented breast cancer—thus linking hormones to cancer.[5] In 1940 Higgins showed that lives of patients with prostate cancer could be prolonged with estrogens. Later many studies on DES (DiEthylStilbestrol), post-menopausal estrogens and steroids have shown their relationship to a number of cancers of target organs like breasts, uterus and ovaries.

In 1925 research in laboratory animals showed that vitamins, especially A, could protect the body from cancer. In 1960 interest in the role of diet in the causation of cancer revived. Fats were found to be promoters of cancer, especially of uterus, ovaries, prostate, and colon. The role of alcohol in cancer causation is becoming more clear. Some food additives like food colors have been implicated in the causation of cancer and subsequently banned.

Recent studies on air, water and pollution of the food chain have shown a relationship with cancer. This area is covered in more detail in Chapter 10.

POCKETS OF CANCER WORLDWIDE

It has been shown that a number of environmental agents can cause cancer. This finding is supported by studies in cancer patterns and cancer "hot spots" around the world.

Internationally, the wide variation in the distribution of cancer is easily explained on the basis of environmental exposures. For example, in countries where tobacco smoking rates are high, incidence of tobacco-related cancers is correspondingly high. Lung cancer rates are highest in Scotland, followed by the United States and Portugal—countries with the highest smoking rates. Similarly, cancers of the breast, prostate, uterus and colon can be considered cancers of affluence; they occur most frequently in the Western countries which consume a diet high in animal fats. The rates of these cancers are lower in Asian countries, well-known for their diets low in animal fat. In third world countries liver cancer is the killer. The Japanese struggle with stomach cancer, according to Dr. John Cairns, a researcher at Harvard University.[6]

This variation in the cancer rates is also seen nationally and locally. Comparison of cancer rates in different parts of the United States shows that bladder cancer rates are highest in New Jersey, where most of the petrochemical industries and toxic dumps are located. Lung cancer rates are higher in coastal Virginia and Florida where there are high levels of asbestos exposure from shipyards. On the other hand, Mormons in Utah experience half the cancer rates of the rest of the country; they consume a low fat diet, with more fruits and vegetables, and are prohibited from use of tobacco and alcohol by their religious beliefs.

There are many examples of cancer clusters on the local level. Grand Junction, Colorado, had unusually high cancer rates. It was found that radioactive tailings had been used as land fill in the area, putting home owners at the highest risk for lung cancer. There have been a number of instances where asbestos or benzene workers have carried pollutants home, increasing their families' cancer risk.

STUDIES OF MIGRANT POPULATIONS

The migration of people from one country to another can be likened to an unplanned experiment conducted on human beings. Here we see a total change in the environment, and migrants have been shown to

3

adopt the cancer rates of their new homeland. For example, Scandinavians who moved to Australia have rates of malignant melanoma similar to local Australians from the excessive exposure to sunlight. Another example can be seen among Japanese who have moved to the United States. Japanese living in Japan are at a high risk for stomach cancer and at a low risk for colon cancer compared to rates for people living in the United States. William Haenszel of the National Cancer Institute and Minoru Kurihara of Tokuhu University School of Medicine in Sendai, Japan found that rates of stomach cancer in Japanese go down and rates of colon cancer go up when they change their eating habits from the traditional high fiber Japanese diet to an American diet much higher in animal fat.[7]

HIGH AND LOW RISK PEOPLE

Cancer risk can also be determined by the intensity of carcinogenic exposure within an environment. Certain occupations can put many people at higher risk for cancer because of the intensity of exposure to cancer causing agents. For example, smokers have 10-20 times the risk of getting lung cancer as compared to the general population, but an asbestos worker who smokes is at 90 times the risk of getting lung cancer! Dye workers are at high risk for bladder cancer and petrochemical workers are at greater risk of brain and kidney cancers. Many other work situations put people at increased risk by exposure to chemicals or radiation.

On the other hand, non-smokers and non-drinkers comprise the low risk populations who have much lower rates of cancer.

SEX DIFFERENCES

While men picked up the smoking habit during World War I, women became smokers later, during World War II. Consequently, while the rate of lung cancer in men has been increasing steadily, rates for women are catching up quickly. The cliche, "You've come a long way, baby!" is proving true; as more women live like men, more women die like men.

AGE DIFFERENCES

There are two peaks in cancer rates, one in infancy and childhood, and the second in old age. The peak during infancy and childhood reflects the environment "in utero." There are many examples where tobacco, alcohol and drugs like DES and Thalidomide have crossed the placental barrier and affected the fetus. Many childhood cancers may be

4

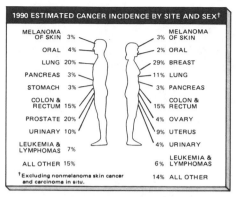

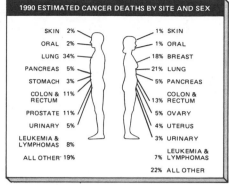

Cancer Statistics 1990
Reprinted with permission from *Ca-A Cancer Journal for Clinicians* Vol.40, No.1, Jan/Feb 1990

related to the mother's use of cigarettes or alcohol during her pregnancy. Similarly, in old age the cancers can be related to cumulative exposures to carcinogenic agents throughout a lifetime. The probability that a man will develop cancer in the next five years is one in 700 at age 25, and increases to one in 14 by age 65—nearly 50 times greater a risk. Dr. Robert Peto and his associates found that animals have exhibited similar tendencies.[8]

From the above evidence, it can be seen that cancer is a generic name given to 200 diverse diseases which have different causes. Most causes are in our environment, in our air, water, food, and working and living areas. Eighty to 90 percent of cancers are caused by environmental factors—factors which are to a large extent controllable, and therefore preventable.

WAYS TO PREVENT CANCER: A Three Pronged Approach

Primary Prevention: Since many carcinogenic agents have been identified, we can educate people on how to avoid them. Such measures are to offer treatment to those trying to quit smoking, preventing exposure to second-hand smoke, encouraging dietary improvements and restricting the use of alcohol. We can also minimize the exposure to radiation and sunlight. Active effort can also be made in terms of AIDS, hepatitis B and elimination of genital warts. Also, we can work to clean up the environment to assure clean air, water and food. All practical steps can be taken to minimize the exposure to chemicals at home and in the workplace. Some educational programs are being started in educating the public about cancer prevention.

Secondary Prevention: Early detection of cancer is generally associated with higher cure rates. The use of Pap smears for cervical cancer and mammograms for breast cancer have been found to greatly increase the success rates for cures. Programs designed for early detection of skin, prostate and colon cancer are catching up fast. Patients with a family history of cancer or hereditary cancer should be checked frequently by screenings and regular examinations.

Tertiary Prevention: Adequate treatment of the cancer patient is necessary to prevent recurrence. The saying goes that "once a cancer patient, always a cancer patient," so careful follow-ups are critical.

Sadly, preventative medicine is not paid for by medical insurance companies. The benefits of prevention can not be demonstrated in the dramatic or statistical fashion of cancer cures. Furthermore, physicians are seldom as well-trained in the philosophy of preventing disease, and have little incentive for such prevention, as they are in the arts and skills of treating and healing ailments already present.

For successful cancer prevention, both education and legislation are necessary for control and regulation of the above three-pronged approach. Dr. Donald Gemson of the Columbia School of Public Health feels that educational programs should be started in the community, work place and school health education programs—and last but not least, that all physicians should be better trained and have greater incentives for the prevention of cancer.[9]

CHAPTER ONE NOTES

1. K. Yamagiwa, and K. Ichikawa, *Journal of Cancer Research*, (1918)

2. G. M. Findlay, *Lancet*, (1928)

3. Howard P. Rusch, et. al. *Archives of Pathology*, (1941)

4. Peyton Rous, *Journal of Experimental Medicine*, 13:397, (1911)

5. Lathrop and Loeb. *Raven* RW: Cancer, Vol. 1., p.5, (London: Butterworths, 1957)

6. John Cairns, *Nature Magazine*, (January 1981)

7. William Haenszel, and Minoru Kurihara, *Journal of National Cancer Institute*, (January 1968)

8. Robert Peto, et. al. "Cancer and Aging in Mice and Men," *British Journal of Cancer*. 32:411 (1975)

9. Donald Gemson, *New England Journal of Medicine*, (March 19, 1987)

CHAPTER TWO

BIOLOGY: HOW DOES A CANCER START?

NORMAL CELLS

There are five billion to one trillion cells in the human body. That number comes to thirteen digits on your calculator. These cells are the building blocks of human life; if any one of them goes awry, a cancer can develop. Even though we see new cases of cancer every day, there is also a miraculous capacity of the human body to resist its formation. Fortunately, cancers can be considered a rare occurrence.

In this chapter we will examine the workings of a normal cell with its sets of external and internal controls. These keep the normal cell in check at all times: telling it when to rest or when to multiply.

When a cell has been damaged it first loses its external controls, in part or in full, and then the internal controls become defective. The result is that the cell must attempt to develop a new set of internal controls for itself. It goes out of sync and starts multiplying at a rapid pace, leading to cell accumulation and the formation of colonies throughout the body.

A normal cell is like a fortress with many internal factories and a great communication network. Simply put, a cell has three components: the cell wall, the cytoplasm, and the nucleus.

Cell walls or cell membranes are made out of carbohydrates, protein and fats, and have the function of maintaining the cell's integrity. These cell walls protect the cell from physical, chemical, or infectious invaders, but when they become defective or weak—through such factors as vitamin A deficiency—chemicals are able to penetrate the cell readily and cause cancer. An example is the case of smokers who also show vitamin A deficiencies. They are at higher risk for lung cancer. Smokers who have been put on high vitamin A intake reduce their risk. Cell walls also have the important function of communicating with the rest of the body through dietary, hormonal and immune system controls.

Between the cell wall and the nucleus is the cytoplasm, the main factory of the cell. The cytoplasm contains fluids with messenger proteins such as Ribonucleic Acid (RNA).

The nucleus contains a nucleic acid called Deoxyribonucleic Acid (DNA). It has many enzymes and chemicals that are needed for the cell's normal functioning. The nucleus is the cell's blueprint. It contains chromosomes which are like rolls of twisted stepladders. There are 23 pairs of chromosomes in the nucleus: 22 that determine the individual's physical traits and characteristics, and one pair for the determination of sex. There are specialized areas on these chromosomes, called genes, which are just like beads on a string.

There are approximately 50,000 genes in our body. With the aid of new DNA recombinant technology over the last decade, many of these genes have been identified and studied. What is more, researchers have been able to study the functions of these minuscule particles encoding life in the laboratory.

Some of the genes with highly specialized functions are called oncogenes. At first, because so many of these genes were seen in different cancers, they were wrongfully labelled "cancer genes." We now know better; oncogenes are extremely important for normal cell division, growth, and maturity and also for their specialized performance of different functions in the body. Oncogenes also direct the repair and replacement of damaged cells by manufacturing necessary proteins. They make this process very accurate, orderly, and precisely controlled. These genes have been preserved in the animal kingdom for millions of years, showing that they are vital to our existence and to the preservation of life itself. A more appropriate name for them is "growth genes."

During our lifetime, the cells in the skin and bone marrow continue to divide and replace old cells. They are always in some portion of a growth phase, in contrast to cells in the rest of the body which are in a resting phase. Whenever a need arises for a certain area to be repaired, neighboring cells move into the growth phase and multiply to repair the damage. When a cell divides in two, "daughter" cells result. These daughter cells grow, mature and specialize under the direction of oncogenes, and finally go into a resting phase.

WHAT HAPPENS TO CHANGE NORMAL CELLS?

What happens when the DNA of a cell is exposed to a physical or a chemical insult? Heat, radiation, chemicals in tar compounds and pesticides, as well as infection by viruses, are some examples of "insults." In such an event, two things can happen to the cell: (1) If the insult is too great, the cell will die outright, a lethal insult; or (2) If the insult does not kill the cell, it becomes a sub-lethal insult, and two more things can happen. The cell can either fully repair the damage to the DNA and become a completely normal cell, or, the DNA becomes permanently altered from the initial damage or from faulty repair. The latter is called a "mutation," a process that cannot be reversed. The consequence of the damage to the genes involved in mutation will depend upon the function performed by those particular genes.

In general, chromosomes are constantly breaking off and rearranging themselves. These breaks are more likely to happen at the weak spots on the chromosomes called "fragile sites." Michael Gold observed that everyone has some of these, but some people inherit more fragile sites than others, and that makes them more vulnerable to cancer.[1]

Dr. Dennis J. Slamon of UCLA School of Medicine explains two major mechanisms involved in converting a normal growth gene into an abnormal one. The first mechanism is a change in the structure of the gene itself, resulting in abnormal gene products. The second is a change in the controls of these genes, causing them to create excessive amounts of gene products.[2]

Cancer does not occur overnight. In most situations, cancer develops over a long, drawn out, multi-step process that goes on for as long as 30 to 40 years after exposure to a cancer-causing agent. Dr. David Schottenfeld, Chairman of the Public Health Department at the University of Michigan Medical School, describes it as a "self-perpetuating program error" in the DNA of the nucleus of the damaged cells.[3]

THE TWO HIT THEORY: INITIATION AND PROMOTION

In 1971, Dr. Alfred Knudson proposed a "two hit" theory for cancer; the first hit defined as initiation and the second hit as promotion. The following explanation is written according to the biology of cancer as described by Drs. Robert E. Scott, John J. Wille, Jr. and Marjorie L. Wier.[4]

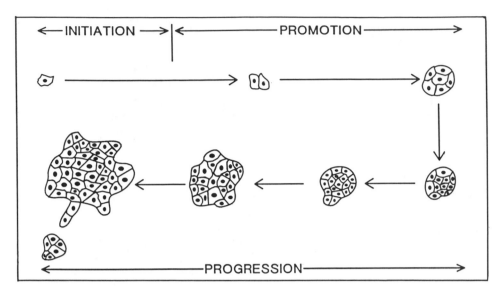

Initiation and Promotion of Carcinogenesis
Reprinted, by permission, from the Mayo Clinic Proceedings, February 1984, p.108, Vol.59

Mutation is the first step in this process, and is called the initiation or first hit. After mutation, the cell is primed and ready to be molded like hot iron by the second hit: promotion. It is at this point that a normal cell is changed into a cancer cell. This cancerous cell then progresses, multiplies, and spreads—sometimes to other parts of the body.

In the first stage of initiation, the cell has been hit and permanently damaged. It is a quick process that can be hereditary or acquired. If the first hit is hereditary, the second hit will come from the environment, as in the case of abnormal moles (dysplastic nevus) which can turn into malignant melanoma when exposed to sunlight. In most cancers, both "hits" come from the environment. For example, some people who chew tobacco have white patches in their mouth. This condition, called leukoplakia, leads to cancer of the mouth. Similar situations exist in people with genital warts, which become cancerous. This evidence suggests that if you can detect the initiated cells early enough, you could prevent cancer from forming. For example, an early Pap smear can diagnose cancer of the cervix.

Initiation, then, can be brought on by environmental factors like chemicals, radiation or infections and in a small number of cases by heredity.

Promotion is the second hit and can occur only with cells that have been primed. In other words, the iron has to be hot before you can hit it and mold it into different shapes and objects. Promotion is a continuous march toward the formation of cancer. Here the initiated cell has come out of the resting phase and has been jolted into a series of rapid, uncontrolled cell divisions. Either fully or partially, the cell has lost its external and internal controls set by the body. To compensate, it has developed its own set of controls and has become an autonomous body. An analogy might be a teenager who has dropped out of school (initiation) and then steals a gun and is ready to commit crimes (promotion).

Unlike initiation, which is a quick and permanent hit, promotion is a much slower process which stretches out over many years. It can also be reversible in its early stages. This is turning into an area of important and exciting research called chemoprevention. Carotenoids (vitamin A precursors) have been used to reverse the promotion stage. Vegetables in the mustard family contain chemicals called anticarcinogens or cancer inhibitors which can interfere with promotion. These will be discussed in later chapters.

The early stage of promotion can be influenced by many factors, including diet, hormones, and infections. For example, female and male hormones can make the conditions favorable for growth of hormone dependent cancers, especially in the area of reproductive organs. Dietary factors such as vitamin A and vitamin C interfere with this stage of promotion. Alcohol can act as a promoter also, either by itself or in tandem with tobacco. Similarly the genital wart virus could cause cancer of the cervix and penis more frequently in smokers (described later in the section on contagious cancers, Chapter 8). Viruses and chemicals can interact to cause cancer. For example, aflatoxin and alcohol damage the liver and Hepatitis B causes liver cancer.

PROGRESSION

Progression is the final stage before the cancer spreads. This period is also long, usually 10-15 years. Here the cancer becomes fully developed, and how fast it progresses depends to a great extent on the aggressiveness of the tumor. The more immature the cells are, or the less differentiated, the faster they tend to progress. Mature cells will progress slower. To some extent the progression of the cancer also depends on dietary factors, hormones, and the individual's immune system.

If the immune system is depressed, as in cases of AIDS, the AIDS related cancers like lymphomas and Kaposi's sarcoma develop and tend to spread quickly. If the immune system is active, it can still eliminate the cancer completely, as in cases of melanomas where spontaneous regression has been known to occur. Studies of "immune enhancers"

11

such as Interleukin-2 and Interferon—which eliminate cancer by boosting the immune system—is a very promising area of drug research.

Hormones are also being used as cancer inhibitors. In cases of breast cancer, anti-estrogen medications are being used to make conditions unfavorable for cancer. Similarly, the female hormone estrogen is being given to prostate cancer patients to prevent the progression of their cancer.

Nutrition still has an important role after cancer is established. Starvation has even been used as a way to shrink tumors. New studies in the area of vitamins show that they have tremendous anti-cancerous powers.

There are many stages in the progression of cancer, allowing time for interference. Early detection of cancer is important for this reason. Many cancers follow the same stages, but I will use the example of cancer of the cervix for illustration. Dysplasia, or an abnormality of the cervix which can lead to cancer, can be detected by a Pap smear. Dysplasia is classified into stages I, II, III, etc., indicating the stage of progression. Vitamin A derivatives called retinoids have been known to reverse dysplasia in the cervix, and also the patches in the mouth called Leukoplakia, mentioned earlier.

In-situ or pre-invasive cancer describes situations where cancer has developed but is localized in the lining of the particular organ. In the case of cervical cancer, the cancer would be localized in the uterus where it could be surgically removed by a procedure called conization of the cervix.

Invasion is the final stage of progression. Here the tumor cells go deeper than the lining of the organ—into the surrounding tissues—but are still localized. Nonetheless, this stage of cancer is extremely serious, as it can easily lead to a spread of the cancer, or metastases.

METASTASES

Metastases is the final stage of cancer development, where cancer cells have spread throughout the body through blood vessels or lymphatic channels and set up colonies in different and unrelated organs, invading the tissues, and eventually killing the host.

TERMINOLOGY

Terms commonly used in discussions about cancer can be confusing. Simple definitions of terms, such as the types of cancer or cancer causing agents, are listed in the glossary in the back of the book, page 254.

1. Michael Gold, "Cancer: When Chromosome Breaks." *Science*, (Sept. 1983)

2. Dennis J. Slamon, *New England Journal of Medicine*, (Oct. 8, 1987)

3. David Schottenfeld, "Genetic and Environmental Factors in Human Carcinogenesis," *Journal of Chronic Diseases*, 39:12 (1986)

4. Robert E. Scott, John J. Wille, and Marjorie L. Wier, "Mechanisms for Initiation & Promotion of Carcinogenesis: A Review and a New Concept," *Mayo Clinic Proceedings*, 59:107-117, (1984)

Chapter Three

TOBACCO

INTRODUCTION AND HISTORY

The cigarette industry in the United States is a 33 billion dollar a year industry and is even larger world wide. It ranks among the top five industries in the United States in terms of assets. According to Drs. Nancy A. Rigotti of Harvard University and Luther Terry,[1] the use of tobacco persists despite the warnings of the United States Surgeon General; despite responsibility for two and one half million deaths each year worldwide—390,000 in the United States alone; despite the publication of more than 30,000 research papers throughout the world showing tobacco as the main factor in illnesses ranging from cancer to emphysema and cardiovascular diseases; and despite the increasing risk of cancer in the general public from second hand smoke in public places where smoking has not been well controlled.

Tobacco, in spite of its hazards and risks, has become firmly entrenched in the economic framework of our society. The total annual contribution of tobacco to the national economy, including spin-off industries, is about *60 billion dollars*. It provides the federal, state, and local governments with more than six billion dollars in tax revenues, and employs two million people (about 2½ percent of all private sector jobs) in the United States. In 1982 more than 623 billion cigarettes were sold to 55 million consumers.[2]

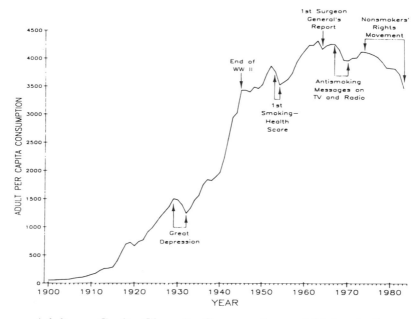

Adult per Capita Cigarette Consumption and Major Anti-Smoking Events Reprinted by permission from *The New England Journal of Medicine*, Vol.3/2 #6, P.387, 1985

Smoking started to catch on in the early 1900s, increased in use during the First and Second World Wars, and peaked in 1955 when half of the American male population were smokers. By the Second World War women, too, had begun smoking in large numbers. The rate started decreasing in 1964 at the time of the Surgeon General's report affirming the health hazards of smoking.

Dr. Michael C. Fiore and his associates at the Center for Disease Control state that there are presently 50 million American adult smokers over age 20; this constitutes about 32 percent of the male and 27 percent of the female population. It is estimated that nearly 4,000 American children take up smoking every day. Teenagers also smoke in large numbers. In one high school senior class in 1977, 30 percent of the girls and 25 percent of the boys smoked; by 1984 the percentage had dropped to 20 percent of the girls and 16 percent of the boys. However, the rate of initiation is higher for females, while the rate for quitting smoking is higher for males.

Fortunately the prevalence of smoking in the general population is declining at the rate of one percent yearly, and at a faster pace for men than women. It is estimated that by the year 2000 only 22 percent of adult Americans will smoke (approximately 40 million people).[3]

REAL COSTS OF SMOKING

DID YOU KNOW THAT?

- Smoking costs over 100 billion dollars yearly. Most of these costs are paid by non-smokers.[4]

- Over 35 billion dollars a year is spent in America on medical care for people with smoking related diseases (50 percent for cardiovascular, 30 percent for emphysema and other respiratory disease, and 20 percent for lung cancer) of which the federal government pays billions in the form of Medicare/Medicaid (1985 statistics).[5]

- According to the United States Fire Administration, there were over 300 million dollars in property damage from fires caused by cigarettes in 1981, and 65,000 fires were started by the careless handling of burning cigarettes.[6]

MARKETING TOBACCO

The use of tobacco in the United States has its origins as far back as the very first Americans. American Indians burned tobacco regularly in campfire ceremonies and celebrations. They smoked through their nostrils, using a special pipe whose long thin tube was called a "tobago" —from which the word "tobacco" was derived.

The nicotine in the fumes that were emitted created a terrific "high." This pleasure was first reported in Europe by Christopher Columbus and his crew when they returned from their American adventures. They were first exposed to tobacco within 24 hours after landing, when they were made welcome and entertained by the American Indians.

One hundred years later, Sir Walter Raleigh saw the business potential in the product. He had the Virginia colonists cultivate the crop while he promoted its benefits throughout England, building a market for the fledgling industry.

King James I, England's reformist king, despised the habit and was said to have had the first known "No Smoking" sign displayed prominently in his private elevator. The king ultimately had Raleigh beheaded for a variety of unsavory activities, but he could not stem the accelerating use of tobacco throughout Europe.

In 19th century America, the widespread popularity of chewing tobacco brought with it further health hazards. Public spittoons were found to be breeding grounds for all sorts of respiratory diseases, especially tuberculosis.

Technology kept up with the public's increasing awareness of sanitation and hygiene, and by 1884, as the practice of chewing and spitting tobacco came under attack, the first automatic cigarette rolling machines were installed in tobacco factories in Virginia. Mass production of cigarettes began, making cigarette smoking accessible to everyone.

Mass production combined with mass marketing propelled tobacco to the top of the money-making agricultural products. But the economic opportunities for this industry, predicated on leisure and pleasure, had just begun.

HEALTH PROBLEMS EMERGED QUICKLY

In later decades of the 20th century, as research about effects of tobacco smoke became more advanced, many health problems were found to be linked to smoking. The first and foremost problem was nicotine addiction. A secondary problem, but no less serious, was the damage caused by the additives in cigarettes. Low tar cigarettes did not live up to their promise of decreasing smoking related illnesses and in fact, only served to make things worse. Health problems were not limited to those doing the smoking; innocent bystanders caught in the deadly side stream of environmental tobacco smoke were also affected.

4,000 COMPOUNDS PER PUFF

It is deceiving to call the blue filmy smoke from a burning cigarette simply "tobacco smoke." The smoke is not pure nicotine, but smoke full of lethal chemicals and radiation particles leading to illnesses, disabilities and hundreds of thousands of deaths annually. Chemical analysis of this smoke shows that it is made of 4000 individual compounds. Where do these chemicals come from? Some of them occur naturally in tobacco leaves. Some are produced while preparing tobacco for consumption. Others are additives and contaminants, and still others are produced when the tip of the cigarette burns at a temperature of 1900°F.[7]

The cultivation of delicate tobacco plants requires a great deal of fertilizer and approximately 18 applications of pesticides. The pesticide residues stay on the tobacco plants even after harvesting. When the tobacco leaves mature, they contain concentrated amounts of radiation particles from the high phosphate fertilizer, along with the tar compounds they produce naturally. When these leaves burn, not only are these compounds released, but many other compounds are formed by the heat of the fire.

The cigarette smoke that is generated is a mixture of particles and gases. These particles are a mixture of nicotine, tar, radiation and various other substances. The gases are a mixture of nitrosamines, formaldehyde, volatile polycyclic hydrocarbons, vinyl chloride, and acrylonitrile (used in making plastics).

Among the particles, there are many tar compounds including benzopyrene, which are known cancer causing chemicals. Nitrosamines found in the smoke are also known carcinogenic chemicals. There are several hundred times more nitrosamines present in smoke than are allowed by the Food and Drug Administration in consumer products. Carcinogenic dyes and heavy metals like nickel, cadmium, and arsenic are also found in cigarette smoke. The radiation particles are more serious; smokers get as much radiation by smoking one and a half packs of cigarettes daily for one year, as they would undergoing 300 chest X-rays, according to estimates by Drs. Thomas Winters and Joseph di Franza of the University of Massachusetts Medical Center.[8] These radiation particles pass through filters and play a very important role in causation of many cancers. With the addition of the pesticide and herbicide residues, the list goes on and on. Smokers are indeed getting a lot for their money!

THE POWERFUL DRUG ADDICTION TO NICOTINE

What happens when a person tries a cigarette for the first time? The physiological changes are not entirely pleasant. He or she may sneeze or cough, get watery eyes or a headache, produce extra phlegm, feel nauseous, have sinus drainage and an increased pulse rate. But within seven seconds of the first puff, the impact of nicotine strikes a chord within the pleasure center of the brain that may take precedence over the superficial unpleasantness.

As early as 1942, a research study by Dr. Lennox M. Johnston reported in the *Lancet*, a prestigious medical journal, showed the effects of nicotine. Dr. Johnston injected himself and 35 volunteers with small amounts of nicotine. The subjects consistently reported pleasant sensations, including relaxed muscles, enhanced memory and attentiveness, and even decreased appetites. When he gave his subjects heavier doses of nicotine, they waited longer before smoking again. The researchers concluded that smokers smoked for these pleasant sensations of nicotine the same way opium addicts smoked to achieve the high from morphine.

Nicotine does indeed have the capability of producing this kind of a "high" in smokers. One study showed that smokers scored higher than

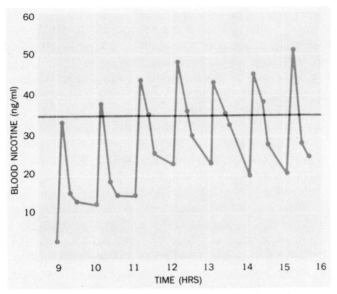

Illustration of smoker manipulating inhalation pattern to get desired blood levels of nicotine. Reprinted with permission from *Science Illustrated*, p. 13, Oct/Nov. 1988.

nonsmokers on tests that measure euphoric effects of amphetamines and morphine. Smokers also report that their "high" was greatest during the first cigarette of the day compared to subsequent cigarettes.

A unique feature of nicotine is that it can act both as a stimulant and as a sedative, and it is all within the smoker's control. Shallow puffing tends to increase alertness, while deep "drags" on a cigarette relax the habitual smoker. The reason for this two-way phenomenon lies in the dose of nicotine and its effect on the neurotransmitters in the brain and muscles. Neurotransmitters conduct the impulses to and from the brain. Low doses of nicotine release these transmitters, making the smoker feel more alert. High doses of nicotine block the flow of the transmitters, causing relaxation.

Thus, nicotine enters the bloodstream and reaches the brain in a "trip" which takes only seven seconds. Nicotine's effects only last from 45 minutes to one hour, but once the pleasure centers of the brain have been triggered, the craving begins. Most smokers have to smoke within two hours to prevent withdrawal. There are longer acting, breakdown products that last in the body's chemistry for up to 18 hours—even though the pleasurable effects have disappeared. For example, a

19

pack-a-day smoker puffing on one cigarette for ten puffs gives his/her brain more than *70,000 nicotine shots each year.*[9] It is because of this nicotine build-up that an addicted smoker can make it through an eight-hour night's sleep without craving a cigarette.

Considerable research evidence points to nicotine as the reason most people use tobacco. Tobacco users become dependent on the nicotine and cannot stop smoking. Nicotine is highly addictive and is the most common type of drug addiction. Dr. Joseph di Franza reports that it kills one in four Americans annually.[10] Before 1964 many researchers disagreed on whether nicotine was addictive or not, citing the fact that it produced no withdrawal symptoms, that smokers did not develop a tolerance or act antisocial. But Dr. Michael A. H. Russell, a senior lecturer and consultant psychiatrist at the Addiction Research Unit of Maudsley Hospital in London, has done research on nicotine addiction and reviewed it as a drug in *Drug Metabolism Reviews* (1978). He believes that nicotine should be labelled as a powerfully addictive drug. Similar views have been given by Dr. Neil Benowitz of the Clinical Pharmacology Unit of the University of California in San Francisco.

Since that time our understanding of addictions has improved. There are now four criteria to addiction, and nicotine addiction through smoking meets every one: 1) an initial stage of experimentation followed by escalating use; 2) progressively increasing tolerance and dependence; 3) quitting causes a change in body chemistry leading to withdrawal symptoms; and 4) lack of availability leads to anti-social behavior.

Smokers do develop a tolerance to and dependence on nicotine over time, much as alcoholics develop a tolerance to alcohol. An initiate does not start smoking two packs on his or her first day of smoking. The number of cigarettes smoked in a day increases gradually. Nicotine dependence develops quickly, say Drs. Harold Kaplan and Benjamin Sadock, renowned psychiatrists at the New York University School of Medicine. In their work *Synopsis of Psychiatry*[11] they explain that nicotine is so addictive that 85 percent of those who smoke one cigarette will go on to become regular smokers. They add that nicotine withdrawal syndrome starts within 90 to 120 minutes of the last cigarette smoked and reaches a peak in the first 24 hours after quitting.

Once addicted to nicotine, quitting smoking is so difficult that 80 percent of smokers who quit relapse over a period of the first two years. This relapse rate, as shown in the following illustration, is similar to the rate in heroin addicts and alcoholics. Use of nicotine gum is helpful in the same way use of methadone helps heroin users. Eighty percent of smokers who quit say they have "intense cravings" for cigarettes. They feel tense and irritable, restless and depressed, become confused, and find it difficult to concentrate. Certain physical changes become evident:

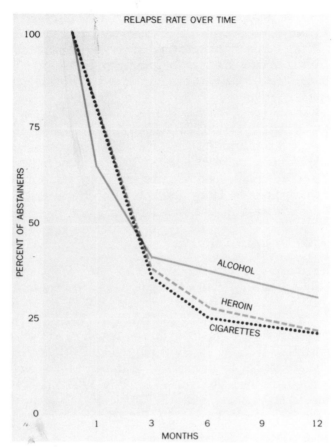

Smokers trying to quit backslide about as frequently as alcoholics and heroin addicts attempting to abstain.
Reprinted with permission of *Science Illustrated*, p. 13, Oct/Nov. 1988

their pulse rates and blood pressure may drop, they complain of constipation, sleep disturbances and difficulty completing simulated driving tests. Drowsiness and headaches have been reported, as have weight gains. All these are symptoms of the "nicotine withdrawal syndrome," according to the American Psychiatric Association.[12]

The withdrawal syndrome is at its highest intensity within 24-48 hours after quitting smoking and gradually decreases in intensity over a period of two weeks. But the desire to smoke continues for years. As shown in the graph, smokers have as much trouble staying off cigarettes as alcoholics do from alcohol and heroin junkies from heroin.

One of the last characteristics of addiction is displaying anti-social behavior. As long as smokers are able to smoke cigarettes, they are not anti-social. If prevented from smoking, they will sometimes resort to extremes. During World War II, for example, German soldiers were known to cheat, steal, trade food rations and even prostitute themselves for a cigarette.

Cigarette smoking has been officially established as an addiction problem. The American Psychiatric Association has acknowledged that nicotine is addictive and physicians today are more often diagnosing cigarette smoking as a cause of death.[13] The Surgeon General's 1988 report has described nicotine as addictive as heroin. Dr. William Pollin of the National Institute on Drug Abuse firmly believes that nicotine is six to eight times more addictive than alcohol.[14]

DEATHS AND DISABILITIES

Cigarette smokers who smoke one to two packs daily have an overall reduced life expectancy of five to eight years. This equates to losing an average of 5½ minutes of life per cigarette smoked, according to Dr. Jonathan Fielding of the University of California. The difference in the life expectancy that we see among male and female senior citizens may very well have to do with the difference in smoking patterns of 30 to 40 years ago. There are more deaths due to tobacco now among male seniors because more men smoked in the early 1900s. Large numbers of women picked up smoking in the 1950s and 60s. Overall, tobacco is responsible for 30 percent of the 412,000 total cancer deaths in United States.[15]

There are more than 350,000 smoking-related deaths each year. The Center for Disease Control estimates smoking-related deaths as 30 percent of the total annual deaths in the United States.[16] This annual number is more than all other drug and alcohol abuse deaths combined, seven times more than all annual auto fatalities, more than 100 times all recorded deaths caused by AIDS, and more than all American military fatalities in World War I, World War II and Vietnam put together.[17]

Lung Cancer

Lung cancer is the most prevalent and serious of the cancers with 110,000 cases reported annually, and has the most obvious connection with smoking. The first major study showing a definite link between cigarette smoking and lung cancer was done by Drs. Ernest Wynder and Evart Graham and published in the May 27, 1950 issue of the *Journal of the American Medical Association*. In 1982, the Surgeon General's Report found that at least 85 percent of lung cancer victims can trace the cause of their illness to tobacco addiction. A study done by Drs. Richard Stevens and Suresh Moolgavkar of the Fox Chase Cancer Center in Philadelphia showed that smokers are at approximately ten times the risk of developing lung cancer.[18]

Another aspect of lung cancer statistics worthy of study is an examination of which groups of people are on an ascending scale. Currently, lung cancer diagnoses have been showing dramatic increases in females and non-white males. In women, lung cancer rates rose from 9.7 deaths per 100,000 women in 1968 to 24.5 deaths per 100,000 in 1982. Lung cancer has overtaken breast cancer as the number one cancer killer among women.[19]

Many famous people have died from lung cancer, including Edward R. Murrow, Damon Runyon, John Wayne, Humphrey Bogart, Lillian Hellman, Arthur Godfrey, King George VI and Nat King Cole. Yul Brenner even made a television commercial before his death begging people not to smoke.

Head and Neck Cancers

Other types of cancers have also shown strong links to smoking. Eighty-five percent of head and neck cancers, such as oral, laryngeal and esophageal cancers, have a death rate of 21,000 persons annually.[20] Dr. B. Herity and his associates of the St. Luke's Hospital in Dublin, Ireland, found a 40 times higher risk of cancer in a smoker as compared to non-smokers and a three times higher risk in a drinker as compared to non-drinkers.[21] These two addictions can be a deadly combination.

Bladder Cancer

Each year more than 50,000 Americans will develop bladder cancer or kidney cancer, and about 20,000 of these persons will die of the disease. Nearly 40 percent of these cancers are related to smoking behavior.[22]

Pancreatic and Stomach Cancer

Pancreatic cancer, a particularly virulent form of cancer which is especially hard to detect, will be diagnosed in about 24,000 persons this year, with approximately 22,000 fatalities. Almost 30 percent of these fatalities can be linked to a past history of smoking.

Stomach cancer, with an estimated death rate of 13,800 deaths per year, has also been linked to smoking. Dr. John Hoey of the McGill University in Toronto showed that smokers have an elevated risk of almost five times of developing stomach cancer as compared to non-smokers. This risk escalated to nine times if these smokers also drank alcohol.[23]

Cervical and Breast Cancer

Recent studies have linked tobacco use to increased risk of cancers of the cervix and breast. Research on links to cervical cancer has shown that both nicotine and cotinine, the end product of nicotine, have been found in the cervical mucus of cigarette smoking women. A recent multicenter study done by Dr. Louise Brinton of the National Cancer Institute indicated that smokers had a two times greater risk of acquiring invasive squamous cell carcinoma of the cervix of the uterus than nonsmokers. In addition, those women who quit smoking were at a lower risk of developing cervical cancer than current smokers.

In a similar study, Dr. Martha Slattery and associates at the University of Utah School of Medicine found that heavy smokers are at four times the risk of cervical cancer. In addition, women who regularly spent three hours or more in smoke-filled rooms were at three times the risk of cervical cancer as compared to the unexposed group.[24]

Premenopausal women smokers seem to be at a greater risk for developing breast cancer than their non–smoking friends—up to 2.1 times greater according to Dr. Martin Schechterpin, assistant professor of Clinical Epidemiology at the University of British Columbia.[25]

Leukemia

One type of leukemia, Acute Myeloid Leukemia (AML), has been linked to cigarette smoking. A study done by Dr. Richard Severson, an epidemiologist involved in the Japan-Hawaii Cancer Study, Kuakini Medical Center in Honolulu, showed that one out of three cases of AML could be linked to cigarette smoking.[26]

WHY DON'T ALL SMOKERS GET CANCER?

"Why doesn't everyone who smokes develop cancer?" The answer is that the development of cancer is determined by a number of factors:

1. Dose of cancer causing chemicals,
2. Age at exposure,
3. Nutritional status,
4. Presence of other cancer causing chemicals in the body; and
5. Strength of the immune system.

It appears that the most significant factor is the dose of the carcinogens. Let us say a man smokes and inhales very deeply, holding the smoke in his lungs for a longer time. There is a greater chance that most of the cancer causing chemicals will get deposited in his lungs and circulate throughout his body. Some of them will be metabolized, some expelled, and some will stay in his body. The most important factors here are the number of cigarettes smoked and the number of years of smoking rather than the tar content of the cigarette. The risk of developing a tobacco-related cancer is about the same for smokers who smoke one pack (20 cigarettes) daily for 20 years, two packs daily for ten years, or four packs daily for five years.[27]

Dr. Terry Pechacek, University of Minnesota, believes that smoking four cigars or pipe bowls is approximately equal to ten cigarettes.[28] This figure can be used to estimate the dose of exposure to the carcinogens for pipe or cigar smokers.

The age of exposure to these carcinogens is also an important factor. People of all ages are exposed to cigarette smoke directly or indirectly. Since the metabolic processes in the young are not very well developed, they stand to have a higher chance of developing cancer. That is why smoking during pregnancy may lead to childhood cancers. The earlier one starts smoking, the more exposure one has to the cancer causing chemicals in tobacco—and the greater the risk of getting a tobacco-related disease. In fact, according to the American Cancer Society, children who start smoking early tend to become heavy smokers as adults.[29]

The third important factor is the nutritional status of smokers. Beta-carotene, a precursor of vitamin A, and alcohol are very important. Apparently, cigarette smoke causes localized vitamin A deficiency. Cell walls become weak and cancer causing chemicals in smoke get into the cells and create havoc. Research done by Dr. Saxon Graham and associates at the State University of New York in Buffalo has shown smokers who increase beta-carotene and vitamin C in their diets decrease the rate of tobacco related cancers in the lungs, stomach, and bladder.[30] Once again, alcohol appears to assist the cancer causing chemicals in the cigarette smoke to enter the cells, thereby multiplying the risk of gastrointestinal and respiratory tract cancers.

The fourth factor in cancer causation is the presence of other cancer causing agents. A smoker is normally at ten times the risk of getting lung cancer as compared to the non-smoking public.[31] The risk for developing head and neck cancers can go up to 75 times in smokers who drink alcohol. If asbestos workers smoke, their risk of lung cancer is 90 times that of the general population. Similarly increased rates of lung cancer have been seen in radiation-exposed smokers who work in uranium mines.[32] If a woman has genital warts and smokes, her risk of cancer of the cervix is much higher. Dr. W. Jedrychowski of the

Institute of Social Medicine in Cracow, Poland, reported that living in cities, because of the higher levels of air pollution with cancer causing substances, also increases the risk for developing lung cancer.[33]

The fifth factor is the status of the immune system. In some cancers such as melanoma, a strong immune system can destroy the cancerous cells and completely eliminate the cancer. Problems with altered immune systems, such as with AIDS patients, is discussed in Chapter 8.

LOW TAR, DASHED HOPES

Reports from the Surgeon General about the hazards of smoking first started appearing in 1956, prompted by the studies done in 1950. These reports raised the consciousness of Americans about the links between cancer and tobacco use. The major tobacco companies found they had to defend themselves. This time, health was the issue and the ideas of low tar and low nicotine were the slogans. The new "low tar" cigarettes, they claimed, posed less of a health risk than regular cigarettes.

In their first attempt, the tobacco industry developed special filters to decrease the amount of tar that reaches the mouth. While these lighter cigarettes may filter out certain large particles, they do nothing to stop smaller tar particles, gaseous compounds like radiation particles, carbon monoxide, nitrosamines, and many other cancer causing agents from reaching the mouth. They do not prevent these agents from being deposited in the lungs or getting into the rest of the body.

The second attempt at making low tar cigarettes was achieved with tiny ventilation holes in the filter, surrounded with porous paper wrappers. The purpose was to ventilate the cigarette smoke by an air dilution principle, decreasing the concentration of these particles and other compounds during the gaseous phase. Several studies have shown that often the smokers nonchalantly cover these holes in the filter with their lips or fingers, making their ventilating function practically useless. Even though smoke inhaled directly is somewhat diluted with these devices, side-stream or second-hand smoke is not affected at all.

Some manufacturers, in a third attempt, even changed the composition of the tobacco by adding fillers and flavor enhancers. The charcoal particles added to the common cellulose filter would then separate and remove gases from the vapors and these foreign by-products.

Cigarettes are determined to be low tar on the basis of Federal Trade Commission smoking machines which take a limited number of drags to determine the tar content. This has considerably helped the sales of low tar cigarettes. Two out of every five packages of cigarettes sold in this country each day are a low tar/low nicotine brand. According to the *New York State Journal of Medicine* (1982), sales have gone up from 17 percent in 1976 to 59 percent in 1982.

A number of recent studies have shown that low-yield cigarettes are more dangerous than regular cigarettes. In Connecticut, Dr. J. W. Meigs did a study of cancer in women. He demonstrated that women in the 35-44 year age group, who usually smoked low-tar cigarettes, showed a ten percent higher rate of lung cancer than men in the same group. A similar report showed that smokers of low-tar cigarettes die earlier than smokers of non-filter cigarettes.[34]

Given a cigarette with a filter, what does the resourceful and addicted smoker do? They are able to manipulate the dose of nicotine on a puff-by-puff basis. Compensation is made by taking larger puffs, inhaling more deeply and for longer periods, puffing intensely and more frequently, and smoking more cigarettes. This shows great determination in maintaining the nicotine level in the blood. We know that the danger of smoking-related diseases increases with the number of cigarettes smoked and for the number of years, and not with the kind of cigarettes. Any smoker who is said to maintain a certain nicotine level is deceiving him or herself into believing that the low tar/low nicotine cigarettes will decrease the risk of cancer or any other disease. One study done on inhalation patterns by Dr. Nicholas Wald of the Cancer Epidemiology Unit of the Radcliffe Infirmary in Oxford, England, showed that the people who smoked ventilated filter cigarettes inhaled 82 percent more often than the smokers with plain cigarettes.

New on the market are ultra low-yield cigarettes. It is too soon yet to see how they will affect smokers. They do deliver less nicotine but may end up producing more toxins.

SECOND-HAND SMOKE: GETS INTO MORE THAN YOUR EYES

It may sound like the sentiments in a classic love song, but there is nothing romantic about the effects of inhaling the second-hand smoke from the cigarettes of the person you love and live with, work beside, or sit next to at public places.

Second-hand smoke comes from two sources. First is mainstream smoke exhaled by the smoker, and the second is side-stream smoke which comes out of the burning tip of the cigarette. In a 12 minute burning period, two-thirds of a cigarette's smoke enters the environment as second-hand smoke. Dr. Leonard Seltzer and Judy Seltzer, R.N., found that the smoker inhales the smoke for only 24 seconds.[35] When the cigarette is being smoked, the tip burns at 1900 degrees Fahrenheit; at such a high combustion rate fewer numbers of particles are produced and released. The opposite occurs when a lit cigarette is not being smoked, and burns slowly in the ashtray or as it is held. The chemistry of this second-hand smoke is quite different from the smoke inhaled by the smoker.

Chemistry of Second-hand Smoke

The chemical analysis of second-hand smoke when compared with inhaled smoke reveals that the second-hand smoke contains:

1. Two times more tar compounds;
2. Three and a half times more benzopyrene, the known cancer causing chemical;
3. Fifty-two times more nitrosamines;
4. Sixteen times more naphthalene;
5. Twenty-eight times more methyl naphthalene;
6. Five and a half times more toluene; and
7. Five times more radiation particles than inhaled smoke.[36]

When these carcinogenic chemicals are multiplied so many times, it is little wonder that sitting next to a smoker may make you sick!

Meaning to the Non-Smoking Public

There were many research studies done on light smokers in the 1970s. One by the American Cancer Society and another done in Sweden, both showed that smoking one to nine cigarettes daily would create approximately two to five times the risk of lung cancer.[37] The Surgeon General stated that since there is no safe level of smoking, second-hand smoking began to be considered a health hazard.

One study projects that between 2,500-8,400 of the total of 12,200 deaths each year may be attributable to lung cancer caused from passive smoking—being caught in this deadly sidestream. Even though only 30 percent of adult Americans smoke, more than 50 percent of adults and 70 percent of children live in homes with one adult smoker, according to Dr. Scott Weiss, Associate Professor of Medicine at Harvard Medical School.

The proof of cancer related to exposure of second-hand smoke has been seen both in adults and in children. A study done by Dr. Goran Pershagen and his associates at the National Institute of Environmental Medicine in Stockholm, Sweden showed that adults working an eight hour day with smokers in the room could receive as much second-hand smoke as smoking one to two cigarettes daily. Proof of second-hand smoke at home in causation of cancer has been seen in many studies around the world. There have been a number of studies in Greece, Japan, the United States and Sweden. Most of them found that a non-smoker had a one and a half times higher risk of getting lung cancer if they were married to a smoker than if they lived with another non-smoker.[38] Living with a smoker also increased a non-smoker's risk of developing cervical or breast cancer. Recently the relationship between passive smoking and cervical cancer was confirmed in a study by Dr. Martha Slattery and her associates at the University of Utah School of Medicine.[39] Dr. Slattery found that current smokers have a four times increased risk (at least one pack/daily for five years) and passive smokers are at a three times increased risk for cervical cancer as compared to general population as mentioned earlier.

Similar effects have been seen in children. When they are living in the polluted environment of smokers, they are inhaling cigarette smoke all the time. Even small babies are not spared as they can ingest it through the breast milk of the smoking mother. Dr. Robert Greenberg of the University of North Carolina School of Medicine actually measured the breakdown of products of cigarette smoke in children's urine.[40] Those children who are exposed to second-hand smoke from smoking adults are at much higher risk for respiratory tract infections, bronchitis, pneumonia and more ear, nose, and throat infections. They are irritable and they don't do well in school. Dr. Dale Sandler of the National Institute of Environmental Health Sciences believes that these children also have an increased risk of cancer later in life.[41] Recently two studies have shown that children of smoking parents show twice the risk of dying from leukemia, both as children as well as adults.[42]

Cigarette smokers have ten times higher benzene levels than non-smokers. Gasoline is the main source of outdoor benzene pollution caused by automobiles; the major source of indoor benzene pollution is cigarette smoke.

As in any problem relating to public health, there are two ways it can be handled; through education and legislation. Some suggestions to help deal with the problem of second-hand smoke are given below.

1. It is suggested that when at home, people should smoke outside in the garage or should have a smoke room with a separate ventilation system.
2. Forty-two states in the U.S. have enacted laws relating to public smoking. Smoking has either been banned altogether or is allowed only in designated places. Of course, enforcement of these laws is difficult.
3. Smoking has been banned on airline flights.
4. Separate smoking and non-smoking sections in hospitals, health care facilities, and restaurants do not really help. There should be separate ventilation systems in each section.

THE UNBORN CHILD AND FETAL TOBACCO SYNDROME

Who else is a captive audience to mainstream as well as sidestream smoke? American obstetricians estimate that 25-30 percent of women in this country continue smoking during their pregnancies.[43] These mothers expose the fetus to the horrible chemicals in cigarette smoke through the blood stream into the placenta. Dr. William G. Cohan of the Memorial Sloan-Kettering Cancer Center states that as early as 1935, studies detected an increase in fetal heartbeat and abnormal breathing-like motions, both a sign of fetal distress, as soon as a pregnant woman began smoking a cigarette.[44] In 1957 Dr. W. T. Simpson demonstrated that the offspring of smoking mothers weighed about 200 grams less than those born to mothers who did not smoke, and the rate of premature births among smoking mothers was double that of mothers who did not. These statistics increased proportionately with the extent of the smoking, regardless of socioeconomic status, race, or age. These patterns are also seen in pregnancies complicated by heart disease, anemia, and among women living at high altitudes. From this, obstetricians deduced that decreased oxygen delivery to the fetus was the common feature. Smoking women can cut down the oxygen delivery to the fetus by 25 percent.[45] The placental arteries age prematurely in the fetus of the smoking mother, diminishing the amount of blood and nutrients available to the unborn baby.

The multitude of diseases caused by the smoking mother in a fetus is called "fetal tobacco syndrome." In lab experiments on animals, it has been proven that tobacco smoke is a transplacental carcinogen. There is more than a *50 percent* chance that a child exposed to smoke during the mother's pregnancy will get cancer. Cancers like lymphomas, leukemia, Wilm's tumors, and rhabdomyosarcoma are the common childhood cancers according to Dr. Michael Stjernfeldt of Sweden.[46] The children of mothers who smoke are at up to two times higher risk and the percentage of risk increases as exposure to the cigarette smoke increases. My personal recommendation is that pregnant women should not only refrain from smoking but should avoid all exposure to second-hand smoke.

Going to a bar and having a drink is almost the worst thing a woman can do to her unborn child. The alcohol, an excellent solvent for dissolving chemicals, helps the carcinogenic chemicals in the smoke enter the body. There is a tragic legal question to this problem. Are rights of the unborn being violated?

THE TRAGIC RE-EMERGENCE OF SMOKELESS TOBACCO

There are two common types of smokeless tobacco. The first one is snuff, which is cured ground tobacco and is available as dry snuff, moist, or fine cut. The second is chewing tobacco, which is also available in the forms of loose leaf, plug, or twist chewing tobacco. Snuff is used by putting a pinch between the cheek and the gum or chewing the plug or the leaf. After mixing with saliva, the nicotine is absorbed through the lining of the mouth, goes into the bloodstream and enters the brain.

In the last century smokeless tobacco was criticized because it was found that tuberculosis germs could spread from the saliva in the spittoons. Spittoons were everywhere, just like ashtrays are now. Because of the fear of spreading TB and other infections, smokeless tobacco was discouraged and its consumption dropped sharply by the early 1960s. Consequently cigarettes became more popular and per capita consumption increased from 150 cigarettes per person in 1910 to a high of 4,200 cigarettes per person in the mid-1960s.

Today, cigarettes are under attack because of the dangers of second-hand smoke, which has recreated a market for the dangerous smokeless chewing tobacco. Sales have risen dramatically from 23.7 million pounds in 1978 to 37 million pounds in 1984—a 55 percent increase. Consumer trends show that the popularity of chewing tobacco is progressively increasing at a tremendous rate, at least 11 percent yearly since 1974 according to Robert Abrams, the Attorney General for the State of New York.[47] The Center for Disease Control estimates that there are 22 million users of smokeless tobacco in the United States.

The average user is between 18 to 30 years of age. Unfortunately, the use among teenagers is also very high; an estimated 27 percent of United States male high school students use tobacco. In a study of Oklahoma elementary school children, 13 percent of the boys in the third grade and 22 percent of the boys at fifth grade were using smokeless tobacco.[48] The new studies done on teenagers is even more shocking. A team of dental examiners from the National Institute of Dental Research was sent around the country from school to school in 1986 and 1987. They found that American teenagers using the smokeless tobacco developed white patches in their mouth at a rate as high as 40 percent.[49]

Education of our young children about the dangers of smokeless tobacco is very important to prevent tragedies like the recent death of Sean Marsee. This young athlete died of oral cancer, believed by Dr. Elbert D. Glover to be caused by smokeless tobacco.[50]

The rate of smokeless tobacco use in the United States is really very close to that in India and Pakistan where 30 to 40 percent of the population use smokeless tobacco. These countries have a very high rate of head and neck cancers, almost 40 percent of the total reported cancers of that area.[51] If the use of smokeless tobacco continues in the United States, we can expect the same sort of cancers to increase.

The main reason for the increase in popularity of smokeless tobacco is the tobacco companies' very carefully designed advertisements and promotional campaigns directed at young people. Frequently, smokeless tobacco is endorsed by prominent athletes and rock stars. It is promoted as a "safe substitute" for smoking.

Chemistry of Smokeless Tobacco

Smokeless tobacco causes cancer precisely where it is placed. There is a very interesting story about a 58-year-old Minnesota farmer who placed snuff in his left ear daily or weekly for about 40 years, leaving it there each time for several hours. He developed a skin cancer in the left ear at the site where he placed the smokeless tobacco.[52] Similarly, most of the chewers of tobacco develop a lesion called leukoplakia (white patches in the mouth) which have a tendency to become cancerous in about three to six percent of the population.[53] Women who had used snuff for about 50 years or longer were up to 48 times more likely to have cancer of the mouth compared to non-users.[54]

The main ingredient in smokeless tobacco is the addictive element nicotine. Like cigarettes, it also includes tar compounds, including benzopyrene, radiation particles and nitrosamines. Dr. Gregory Connolly of the Massachusetts Department of Public Health states that the levels of nitrosamines in smokeless tobacco are up to 100 times more than found in cigarette smoke, and 1,400 times more than levels allowed by the Food and Drug Administration and the Department of Agriculture in beer, bacon, and baby-bottle nipples.[55] Also present are pesticide residues and residues of arsenic, nickel, cadmium, and other heavy metals. And the list is not yet finished. Salt and sugar are also added, hazardous to diabetics and patients with high blood pressure, as well as additives and flavoring agents which are "trade secrets."

Dr. P. Grasso gave a written statement to the Massachusetts Department of Public Health Hearings in Boston on February 22, 1985, stating that in experiments on laboratory animals, the nitrosamines found in smokeless tobacco has produced cancer in the mouth, nose, esophagus, and lungs of hamsters and rats. The cancer causing chemicals in chewed tobacco aid other factors in the causation of cancer. One example is Human Papilloma Virus (HPV), the genital wart virus appearing in the linings of the mouth, which is aided by tobacco in causing mouth cancer.

How do you get off this junk? The plan of action is the same as quitting cigarettes.

IF YOU SMOKE — A PLAN OF ATTACK!

One of the most discouraging situations for any physician is seeing the way a patient will cling to a cigarette addiction despite every indication of its destructive effects. Patients are known to come out of bypass surgery, admitted into the intensive care unit for a heart attack, surgery for removal of a cancerous lung, and ask for their cigarettes. Patients in their early 20s with persistent coughs have cried because they cannot give up their smoking addiction, knowing that it does them no good in the short or long term picture for their lives.

It is estimated that 90 percent of adult smokers cannot quit, despite many attempts to do so. Of those addicted to nicotine early in childhood (average age of 13), more than half failed in their efforts to quit and more than one fourth felt they could not quit "no matter what."

Nicotine addiction is very hard for physicians to treat. Before one can quit, it is most important to assess the level of addiction. The Fagerström Nicotine Scale, which follows, can be used as an aid to determine the level of addiction.

Assessment of Addiction

The Fagerström nicotine tolerance scale on the following page has been validated against physiologic measures of nicotine withdrawal, such as body temperature and heart rate changes. Thus, it can be used to assess the extent of nicotine dependency in a specific patient who wants to stop smoking. (Adapted from Fagerström K-O: Measuring degree of physical dependence to tobacco smoking with reference to individualization of treatment.)[56]

Assign no points for each answer in Column A, one point for each answer in column B, and two points for each answer in column C (note that not all questions have an answer in column C). Then, total the number of points to arrive at the Fagerström score. The highest possible score is 11.

Consider patients who score seven or more to be highly dependent on nicotine; patients who score less than six have low nicotine dependence. Bear in mind that a low score does not rule out the use of nicotine chewing gum or other therapy based on physiologic nicotine addiction. In general, however, the higher the score, the better the result of therapy.

THE FAGERSTRÖM NICOTINE TOLERANCE SCALE
(Printed with permission from the Journal of Respiratory Disease).

	A	B	C
1. How soon after you wake up do you smoke your first cigarette?	After 30 min.	Within 30 min.	—
2. Do you find it difficult to refrain from smoking in places where it is forbidden, such as the library, theatre, doctor's office?	No	Yes	—
3. Which of all the cigarettes you smoke in a day is the most satisfying one?	Any other than the first one in the morning.	The first one in the morning.	—
4. How many cigarettes a day do you smoke?	1-15	16-25	>26
5. Do you smoke more during the morning than during the rest of the day?	No	Yes	—
6. Do you smoke when you are so ill that you are in bed most of the day?	No	Yes	—
7. Does the brand you smoke have a low medium, or high nicotine content?	Low	Medium	High
8. How often do you inhale the smoke from your cigarette?	Never	Sometimes	Always

Now that the level of addiction has been determined, we are brought to the issue of exactly how to quit smoking. Dr. M. Therese Southgate describes quitting in three phases.[57]

The first phase is motivation. Motivation is the single most important factor in accomplishing any task in life. Most of the uninitiated think that all it takes to quit smoking is will power, the ability to abstain, to stay away from this messy addiction. However, motivation is a much different issue. It is a deeply held conviction, personal to the individual, to BELIEVE that he/she would be better off without cigarettes than with them. Such thinking about the positive benefits goes beyond the negative, denial aspect of quitting, of doing without something you love and depend upon: in this case cigarettes.

Good motivation can serve as an important anchor once the second phase of quitting, the physical process of withdrawal, wreaks its havoc. Withdrawal entails some days of discomfort. Sleeplessness, constipation, headaches, irritability, unusual cravings for different foods, and mood swings are the most common symptoms of withdrawal from nicotine, but these only last for about a week in their most extreme cases.

The final phase is the most important one—the psychological. Some people experience long term depression or a "grief reaction." I think many people fail in their attempts to give up smoking because their personal motive has not been effectively worked out in the beginning. It is in this phase that most relapses occur.

Of the approximately 37 million people in the United States who have smoked at one time and given it up, about one half have done it "cold turkey"; they have just set a target day and given up cigarettes in one fell swoop! The other half have done it gradually, cutting down the number of cigarettes smoked and even cutting down to lighter, ultra filtered, less flavorful brands as an intermediate step. Add here a diet plan and exercise to fill in the void.

Organized programs, through the work place or religious and community services, as well as private counselling have worked for many people. In my practice, I have used replacement therapy such as Nicorette chewing gum combined with a weekly office visit to help those who wish to quit. Other replacement therapies are in the testing stages.

Nicorette, a nicotine gum, and drugs like Clonidine, used for the treatment of high blood pressure, are commonly used for the treatment of nicotine withdrawal syndrome. Clonidine has been seen to be especially effective in women who are trying to quit smoking. Dr. Michael A. Russell of the Addiction Research Unit at the Institute of Psychiatry in London has found Nicorette to be a very promising replacement therapy in patients who have quit smoking.[58] The Nicorette gum seems to give a nicotine level in the blood which is one-third to two-thirds that of a cigarette and is helpful in blocking the withdrawal symptoms of quitting smoking. In the "quit smoking clinics" the success rate when using Nicorette was 27 percent at six months as compared to 18 percent with a placebo.

Research has shown that Nicorette gum is most effective in highly motivated patients and should be used under physician supervision. The gum is chewed for 20 to 30 minutes when there is an urge to smoke, with a maximum of 30 pieces daily. It should be chewed gently and slowly until a tingling or taste is experienced in the mouth. Chewing should be paused until the tingling or taste disappears. It is better to chew only intermittently as constant chewing can cause jaw fatigue and excessive saliva in the mouth which, if swallowed, cause nausea. One problem with Nicorette gum is that up to 13-38 percent of the patients continue to use it after one year.

New methods to aid quitting are still being created. A new nicotine patch has been developed and, according to a study done in Sweden by Drs. Abelin, Buehler, Müller, this may help one in three patients to quit.[59] Another experimental area is a nicotine nasal spray. The nicotine blood level after use of the nasal spray does appear to be comparative to that achieved by smoking cigarettes. Recently "Favor Smokeless" cigarettes have been released in the United States. These appear to achieve the same blood level as Nicorette chewing gum.

The Buddy System uses techniques developed by the American Lung Association. To begin this program you must set a date about two weeks in advance and think of all good reasons that you want to quit smoking. Start saving cigarette butts in a jar and look at the ugly things frequently when you feel like smoking. Sign a contract with your physician (or a buddy) stating that on the advice of your physician you will stop smoking. Enlist the aid of your spouse or partner. If you succeed in quitting smoking, the partner will be taken on a vacation or given some sort of reward. Buy only one pack of cigarettes at a time instead of an entire carton. Make it hard for yourself to get to them. Remove all smoking paraphernalia from around you. Smoke in the garage instead of the house.

When the set date arrives: drink a lot of liquids and eat lots of fresh fruit and vegetables; arrange low calorie food, less meats, dairy products and fried foods; start a good exercise plan. Weight gain and trouble sleeping will be a problem to be solved, but you will eventually get over these obstacles.

If you are unable to follow this program on your own, go to a hypnotist or join an organized program. The following organized plans are sponsored by the American Cancer Society and the American Lung Association:

> *Fresh Start* (Contact Local Divisions of The ACS)
> *Breaking Free* (Targeted to vocational high school students;
> contact local Divisions of the ACS)
> *Freedom from Smoking* (Contact Local Offices of the ALA)

One interesting approach to quitting is called rapid smoking technique. Relying on the basic principle of aversion therapy, a smoker literally is choked in smoke. Inhaling normally with the supervision of a counsellor or therapist, the smoker takes a drag every six seconds for 10-15 minutes. After about ten sessions, in combination with intensive counselling, the smoker associates smoking with feeling horrible. This method has shown a two year success rate of nearly 50 percent of persons with heart or lung disease.[60]

Women, particularly, worry about weight gain after they quit smoking. Smokers in general weigh five to ten pounds less than non-smokers of similar age and height.[61] One theory to explain the pheno-menon of weight gain is that nicotine dulls the activity of the enzyme lipoprotein lipase, which regulates the storage of fats in the body. When nicotine is not available, this enzyme increases the amount of fats in fat cells. A second theory suggests that nicotine tends to decrease appetite and keeps food in the stomach longer before going to the intestines. In other words, without nicotine, you may feel hungry sooner. A third theory is that nicotine decreases the body's craving for sweets, acting as an appetite suppressant. Cigarette tar actually does form a coating on a smoker's tongue which dulls the taste of food, especially sweets. A fourth theory, based on a report published in the *New England Journal of Medicine* by Dr. Kenneth A. Perkins, shows a 50 percent increase in energy expenditure in smokers by increasing the metabolic rate.[62] No wonder smokers are frequently tired.

Finding other habits to fill up the void left by quitting smoking is essential. This is NOT the time to start a new diet or deprive yourself of anything more that you have come to depend on and enjoy, but why not start a vigorous exercise plan? The continued stress of cigarette smoking on vital organs such as heart and lungs is equivalent to carrying an additional 75 pounds of body weight!

After you've suffered through the physical agonies, how do you know that the campaign has been successful? Most relapses do occur within about three months of successful withdrawal, so don't let your guard down. But recognize, too, that a lapse is not the end, that progress in any area is often a gradual exercise. Two steps forward, one step back. Fortunately, the benefits of quitting are immediate; even if you've smoked for 40 years, the body repairs quickly from the effects.

MARIJUANA

Whether called pot, grass, weed, hashish, *cannabis* or Mary Jane, marijuana is defined by a United Nations Treaty officially mandated in 1969 as "the flowering or fruiting tops of the cannabis plant from which the resin has not been extracted." Marijuana is commonly available in the United States. It is a mixture of the leaves, small stems and flowering tops of the cannabis plant, which are rolled into a "joint" like a hard-rolled cigarette and smoked, or occasionally boiled and served as tea or cooked into foods such as the Alice B. Toklas brownies of literary renown. Instead of tobacco's nicotine, the big lure of marijuana is the mind-altering chemical known as delta 9 THC, an abbreviation for delta tetrahydrocannabinol, which is activated by the heat.

Marijuana has been used for centuries, and current consumption has increased 30 times in the past 20 years. A recent national survey showed that in the United States there are 17.3 million adults and 2.7 million teenagers who smoke marijuana on a regular basis.[63] Another survey done in 1982 showed that 59 percent of high school students had used marijuana at some time in their lives; 35 percent had used it before getting into high school, and six percent of these reported regular use in the previous month.[64]

The chemistry of marijuana smoke is worse than tobacco smoke. All told, there are 421 known chemicals in marijuana. When it is smoked, they burn into 2,000 individual compounds. Except for the active ingredient Tetrahydrocannabinol (THC), the other chemicals are similar to tobacco smoke. However, smoking only a few joints is comparable to smoking 20 cigarettes daily. Tar containing cancer causing chemicals like benzopyrene are 50 percent higher and naphthalene is 70 percent higher in "pot" smoke than in tobacco smoke. The nitrosamine content is the same. Pot smokers are exposed to a very high concentration of pesticide residues because they smoke the stub. Most tobacco smokers stub out their cigarettes before that final half inch that holds the bulk of the toxic and cancer causing chemicals in the most concentrated form. The pot smoker regards the "stub" or the "roach" as the best part of the joint. Roach clips to hold the stub without burning the fingers used to be available in drug paraphernalia stores to make this practice easier. Some marijuana smokers use large pipes called a "bong" or "rush tubes" to smoke more efficiently.

Inhalation patterns are different as well. In fact, pot smokers take puffs twice as large as tobacco smokers, hold smoke 40-50 percent more deeply and retain the smoke in their lungs three to five times longer. The typical tobacco smoker holds the smoke for about two seconds in the lungs. The pot smoker draws the smoke deeper and tries to keep the smoke in as long as possible, from ten seconds to a full minute before exhaling. This keeps the smoke's irritants, the tar compounds, and cancer causing chemicals in the body longer.

Often marijuana smokers believe that their habit does not have the same addictive qualities as tobacco. However, frequent use does build up a tolerance to the drug's effects, and soon more and more potent marijuana is necessary to achieve the same "high."

THC: Effects on the Body

THC is extremely euphoric and addictive. It has been found to be toxic to the immune system and impairs immune system functioning. It has also been linked to cancer. A recent report by Dr. Paul Donald of Sacramento, California, found that some rare head and neck cancers, called Squamous cell carcinoma, have been found in young men who were marijuana smokers.[65]

The National Academy of Sciences formed a committee of experts to review the cancer causing evidence against marijuana. They found that marijuana did cause precancerous changes in the bronchial tubes of smokers similar to those produced by tobacco smoke. Since marijuana smoke has the same components as cigarette smoke, it is suspected to cause lung cancer as well. In laboratory experiments on animals, pot smoke has caused cancers similar to those caused by tobacco smoke. Now, it appears that marijuana smoke may be causing cancers other than ear, nose, and throat cancers, such as bladder cancer.

About ten percent of women smoke pot during pregnancy. It crosses the placenta to reach the fetus and has the same effect in the fetus as fetal tobacco syndrome. It can lead to extremely complicated pregnancies.

Adults or parents of children who need assistance in getting over a marijuana habit may seek help from:

PRIDE (Parents Resource Institute for Drug Education)
   100 Edgewood Avenue, Suite 1261
   Atlanta, GA 30303
   1-800-241-9746

National Federation of Parents for Drug Free Youth
   1820 Franwall Avenue
   Silver Springs, MD 20902
   1-800-554-KIDS

American Council for Drug Education. This organization can be contacted through your local chapter of the American Lung Association.

In addition, there are many publications available which offer information on marijuana and its addictive nature. One book that I highly recommend is *Marijuana Alert* by Peggy Mann.[66]

CHAPTER THREE NOTES

1. Nancy A. Rigotti, "Cigarette Smoking and Body Weight," *New England Journal of Medicine,* (April 6, 1989) and Luther Terry, *New York State Journal of Medicine,* (1983).
2. Chris Kiehne, *Delaware Medical Journal,* (July 1985)
3. *Journal of the American Medical Association,* (Jan. 6, 1989)
4. *Journal of the American Medical Association,* (May 24, 1985)

5. 1985 Statistics, *Environmental Action,* (May/June 1986)

6. John Madeley, "The Environmental Effect of Tobacco Production in Developing Countries," *New York State Journal of Medicine,* (Dec. 1983)

7. *Ibid.*

8. Thomas Winters and Joseph di Franza, "Radioactivity in Cigarette Smoke," *New England Journal of Medicine,* (Feb. 11, 1982)

9. Edward N. Brecher, "Smoking, For the Most Part a Sentence to Nicotine Addiction," *Medical World News,* (March 5, 1979)

10. Joseph Di Franza, *New England Journal of Medicine,* (June 26, 1987)

11. Harold Kaplan and Benjamin Sadock, *Synopsis of Psychiatry,* (Williams & Wilkins, 1988)

12. Similar results were obtained in studies on smokers. *Diagnostic and Statistical Manual of Mental Disorders,* 3rd. Ed. (1987)

13. *Ibid.*

14. William A. Pollin and R.T. Ravenholt, "Tobacco Addiction and Tobacco Mortality," *Journal of the American Medical Association,* (Nov. 23, 1984)

15. *New England Journal of Medicine,* (August 22, 1985)

16. "Smoking and Cancer," *Morbidity and Mortality Weekly Report,* (Feb. 26, 1982)

17. Pollin, "Tobacco Addiction and Tobacco Mortality," *Journal of the American Medical Association,* 252:2874

18. Richard Stevens and Suresh Moolgavkar, *American Journal of Epidemiology,* Vol. 119, (1984)

19. Center for Disease Control. *Journal of the American Medical Association,* (Nov. 23, 1984)

20. *Medical Tribune,* (April 14, 1982)

21. B. Herity, et.al., *British Journal of Cancer,* (1982)

22. *Medical Tribune,* (April 14, 1982)

23. John Hoey, *American Journal of Epidemiology.* Vol. 113, #6, (1981)

24. *Journal of the American Medical Association,* (March 17, 1989)

25. *American Journal of Epidemiology,* (1982)

26. Richard Severson, *Oncology and Biotechnology News,* (September 1987)

27. Neil Martini, *Cancer Consultation,* Vol. 1, No. 1 (1985)

28. Terry Pechacek, "Pipe and Cigar Smokers," *Journal of the American Medical Association,* (Dec. 20, 1985)

29. Pollin, *Journal of the American Medical Association,* (Nov. 23, 1984)

30. Saxon Graham, et.al., *American Journal of Epidemiology,* Vol. 113, #6

31. Rodolfo Saracci, "The Interactions of Tobacco Smoking and Other Agents in Cancer Etiology," *American Journal of Epidemiology,* Vol. 9, (1987)

32. John O'Hara, "Radioactivity in Cigarette Smoke," *New York State Journal of Medicine,* (Dec. 1983)

33. W. Jedrychowski, *Neoplasia,* 30:5, (1983)

34. "Smoking and Health," *New York State Journal of Medicine,* (July 1985)

35. Leonard Seltzer and Judy Seltzer, "Importance of Passive Smoking," *Delaware Medical Journal,* (July 1985)

36. Sandler, *American Journal of Epidemiology*, Vol. 121, #1, (1985)

37. Jonathan Fielding and Kenneth J. Phenow, "Health Effects of Involuntary Smoking," *New England Journal of Medicine*, (Dec. 1, 1988)

38. Francine Kaufmann, Jean Francois Pessier, and Paul Oriol, "Adult Passive Smoking and Chronic Air Flow Limitation in Home Environment," *American Journal of Epidemiology*, vol. 117, #3, (1987)

39. Martha Slattery, et.al. *Journal of the American Medical Association*, (March 17, 1989)

40. Robert Greenberg, et.al., "Measuring the Exposure of Infants to Tobacco Smoke," *New England Journal of Medicine*, (April 26, 1984)

41. Dale Sandler, Richard Everson and Allen Wilcox, "Passive Smoking in Adulthood & Cancer Risk," *American Journal of Public Health*, (1985) 121:1

42. *Medical Tribune*, (January 7, 1987)

43. Cecil Gordon, Jr., "SMoking During Pregnancy," *Delaware Medical Journal*, (July 1985)

44. William G. Cohan, *New York Times*, (1985)

45. *American Journal of Obstetrics and Gynecology*, (1957)

46. Michael Stjernfeldt, et.al., "Maternal Smoking During Pregnancy and Risk of Childhood Cancer," *Lancet,* (June 14, 1986)

47. Robert Abrams, "Attorney General Speaks Out Against Smokeless Tobacco," *New York State Journal of Medicine*, (July 1985)

48. *Medical World News*, (Feb. 10, 1986)

49. Swango, *Medical Tribune*, (May 3, 1990)

50. Elbert D. Glover, *Physician and Sports Medicine,* (Dec. 1986)

51. Council for Scientific American Medical Association, *Journal of the American Medical Association*, (Feb. 28, 1986)

52. Root, *New England Journal of Medicine*, 262:819-20 (1960)

53. Christen, *New England Journal of Medicine*, (April 3, 1980)

54. *New England Journal of Medicine*, (March 26, 1981)

55. *Ibid.* (April 17, 1988)

56. *Addictive Behavior* 3:235-241, (1978)

57. M. Therese Southgate, *Journal of the American Medical Association*, (1986)

58. Michael A. Russell, *Journal of the American Medical Association*, (June 19, 1987)

59. Abelin, Buehler, Müller, *Lancet*, (1989)

60. *Journal of the American Medical Association,* (Nov. 13 1987)

61. Rigotti, *New England Journal of Medicine*, (April 6, 1989)

62. Kenneth A. Perkins, "Effect of Nicotine on Energy Expenditure During Light Physical Activity," *New England Journal of Medicine*, (April 6, 1989)

63. Glasbrenner, *Journal of the American Medical Association,* (Nov.23 1984)

64. Paul Donald, "Marijuana Smoking — Possible Cause of Head & Neck Carcinoma in Young Patients," *Otolaryngology*, (April 1986)

65. *Ibid.*

CHAPTER FOUR

RADIATION, SUNLIGHT AND CANCER

The word "radiation" conjures up various notions—from the nuclear devastation of Hiroshima and Nagasaki, accidents such as Russia's Chernobyl or Three Mile Island in the United States, to the disposal of dangerous nuclear waste products from nuclear reactors, submarines, research facilities, and medical institutions. Stories indirectly related to radiation—the threat of nuclear war or how to harness nuclear energy safely—appear at our doorstep daily with the arrival of the morning newspaper. Just what is radiation, what are its uses, and what is its carcinogenic potential?

There are two basic types of radiation: ionizing and non-ionizing. Ionizing radiation is in two forms of particles and waves. The particles emitted by the nuclear materials are unstable parts of the atoms. The waves emitted by these nuclear materials are called gamma rays. They are produced because unstable electrons inside the atom keep colliding with each other. Similar waves of radiation can also be produced artificially by X-ray machines. The atoms of nuclear materials like radium, thorium, etc., are unstable and restless and emit ionizing radiation in the form of particles and electromagnetic rays. Exposure to ionizing radiation is dangerous because it can damage the nuclear material of the cells of the human body; cancer may eventually form in the area of radiation damage. We are exposed to ionizing radiation in a number of ways: the infamous radon gas, diagnostic and therapeutic radiation, and nuclear materials.

The two types of ionizing radiation in particle form are:

Alpha radiation: The nucleus of heavy elements like plutonium and radon emit particles containing two protons and two neutrons. These can travel over two inches and can be stopped by paper. They can damage cells if they enter the body.

B–radiation: Strontium 90 and Tritium emit streams of electrons travelling at the speed of light. Exposure can be stopped with heavy clothing. B-radiation can cause skin cancer.

One of the latest reports on exposure to ionizing radiation showed that exposure to low-level radiation is three and one-half to five times more dangerous than previously suspected.[1] The average American receives 55 percent of radiation exposure from radon gas. Another 27 percent comes from other natural sources, 18 percent from diagnostic and therapeutic radiology, and less than one-half percent from atomic reactors (primarily affecting workers).

We are also exposed to non-ionizing radiation from many sources like sunlight, sun lamps, televisions, microwaves and video display terminals. This radiation is not as dangerous as ionizing radiation because it does not have the ability to break the chromosome. However, exposure to sunlight has been shown to cause cancer in the skin and eyes.

SUNLIGHT AND CANCER

SUNLIGHT: FRY NOW AND PAY LATER

The slogan above has been made popular by the American Cancer Society, emphasizing that sun and skin are a bad combination. One of the most innocent sources of radiation is sunlight. The sunlight gives off ultraviolet rays which are of three different types, A, B, and C. The ultraviolet C rays called "germicidal rays" are the strongest. These are filtered by the ozone layer surrounding the earth. So ultraviolet rays A and B are the only ones that reach the earth. Of the two, ultraviolet B or "burning rays" are more responsible for skin cancer and wrinkles. Recently, however, ultraviolet A or "tanning rays" have also been incriminated.

The ozone layer is about three millimeters or one-eighth of an inch thick and is present around the earth in the stratosphere within a 15-35 mile zone. This layer is constantly being generated and degraded. Recent research has indicated that air pollution has caused some destruction of the ozone layer. The air pollutants responsible are nitric oxide in aviation exhaust and the increased production and use of CFCs (Chlorofluoro Carbons). CFCs are commonly used as freon in refrigeration and as air propellants. Serious concerns about the safety of this ozone shield around the earth have spurred efforts to ban the production and use of CFCs world wide. It is estimated that every one percent decrease in ozone increases the rate of malignant melanomas by one to one and one half percent.[2]

The earliest links of sunlight to skin changes and skin cancer go back to 1894 and the observations of a German scientist named Paul Unna. By 1928, the connection of sun to skin changes and cancer had been firmly established by Dr. G.M. Findlay.[3] Dr. Harold P. Rusch, Professor of Oncology at the University of Wisconsin, and his associates provided conclusive evidence of the link between ultraviolet light and skin cancer and identified the particular part of the ultraviolet spectrum.[4] Dr. Rusch studied the effects of ultraviolet light on the ears of albino mice, proving that photocarcinogenesis is a continuous and cumulative process that begins with initial exposure and is accelerated by subsequent exposures.

As these rays do not give off much energy, they do not penetrate very deeply into the body. The cancerous effects of ultraviolet radiation appears to be limited to skin cancer and melanoma of the eyes. An overwhelming amount of evidence demonstrates that nearly all skin cancers are due to ultraviolet light exposure. The incidence of skin cancer seems to be increasing dramatically.

More than 500,000 Americans will develop a skin cancer this year; and it is estimated that one out of seven Americans will have skin cancer in his/her lifetime. According to the Skin Cancer Foundation statistics, most of us have received 80 percent of life time sun exposure by age twenty.

Many people are under the impression that skin cancer does not kill. In 1990, non-melanoma skin cancer will claim 2,200 fatalities in the United States alone. Most common are the Basal cell carcinoma or Squamous cell carcinoma. Both of these can be excised surgically and cause little difficulty. While it is true that basal cell cancer does not metastasize through the bloodstream and locate in other parts of the body, if ignored it can dig through the layers of skin and tissue into the bone, and even into the brain. The basal cell cancer can spread in later stages. Squamous cell cancer is the second most common skin cancer in the world's Caucasian population, and the most common cancer in pigmented races. Very closely related to exposure to ultraviolet light, squamous cell cancer is seen more on parts of the skin exposed to sunlight such as the head, neck and extremities. It is therefore less common in people who are protected by high cotton collars, hats, and umbrellas or those with mustaches and beards.

Incidence of skin cancers, both squamous cell carcinomas and malignant melanomas, are rising at an alarming rate. Dr. Andrew Glass of the Center for Health Research at Kaiser-Permanente, Portland, Oregon, and Dr. Robert Hoover of the National Cancer Institute, did a study on the continuous population-based registry of skin cancer cases in the Kaiser-Permanente Health Plan.[5] They found a three to four fold increase in both cancers in men and women between the 1960s to 1980s.

Another type of skin cancer, *malignant melanoma*, is far more deadly, far more aggressive, and fatal 25 percent of the time—despite sophisticated therapies and treatments. It primarily affects caucasians.

Whether due to lifestyle or longevity, the numbers of all three types of cancer have been on the rise. According to the Skin Cancer Foundation, about 25,000 Americans were diagnosed with malignant melanoma in 1989, with approximately 6,000 fatalities.[6] These numbers only give the illusion of being small.

Considered a rare form of cancer just 50 years ago, the Skin Cancer Foundation has the shocking statistic of a rise in the incidence of malignant melanoma by three to four percent yearly, which means that a child born in the 1930s had a lifetime risk of one out of 1,500 of developing a malignant melanoma, while in the 1989 that risk has increased to one in 128. It is expected to reach one out of every 90 by the year 2000![7]

Melanomas used to be thought of only as the result of an existing mole whose cells went haywire. New data relates these skin cancers to ultraviolet overexposure, particularly in childhood, especially among children who are light eyed and have difficulty tanning, and with one or more isolated but blistering and painful episodes of sunburn.

Australia has the highest rate of this disease in the world with 30 cases per 100,000 persons. An Australian study of 511 patients, showed that immigrants arriving before age ten from less sunny areas of the world had the same risk for malignant melanoma as native born Australians. For those who arrived in Australia after age 15, however, the incidence of this disease was only one-fourth as great.[8]

Epidemiologic studies from Norway, Sweden, and Denmark suggest that travel to sunny climates involving short periods of high-intensity sun exposure is also an important risk factor for melanoma. It is this sort of lifestyle that many young professional people living in urban areas of the United States indulge in as well. Recent research has shown that sunlight is not only a risk factor for the cancers of the skin, but also for malignant melanoma of the eye.

Who is at high risk for melanoma?

People with the following qualifications are at the highest risk for melanomas.

1. Blonde hair;
2. Family history of melanoma;
3. Freckling on the back;
4. Actinic keratosis, or sun-damaged skin;
5. Three blistering sunburns; or
6. Three or more outdoor summer jobs as a teenager.

Early Detection of Melanoma

The criteria for early detection were developed by New York University. Most of the dermatologists in this country feel that no one should have to die from melanoma because it is a cancer which is quite unique in that it can be detected early by the patients themselves. The acronym called ABCD has been designed for easy memorization.

A stands for asymmetry. A normal mole is generally symmetrical, which means if you divide a circle into two equal parts both parts are a mirror image of each other. But, melanoma usually grows on one side more than the other, so the lesions are asymmetrical in appearance.

B stands for border. Normally moles have a definite border, but melanomas have a notch in the border due to irregular growth.

C stands for color. Normally most of the moles are uniform in color, but melanomas have color variations. If you see red, white and blue in a mole you should have it checked by your physician.

D stands for diameter. Most moles are usually six millimeters or roughly one quarter of an inch, which is about the size of a pencil eraser, but melanomas are larger than six millimeters in size.

The moles at high risk for turning into malignant melanomas are large flat moles, single dark brown moles and moles present at birth.

A Price to Pay for the Glow of Good Health

There was a time when suntans did not represent leisure, vitality, and an expensive lifestyle. On the contrary, a "lady" at the turn of the century carefully protected her skin with a parasol in the heat of the midday sun, and a tanned body was generally looked upon as the unfortunate result of doing "field work." But styles and trends change. Right now, the incidence of all three types of skin cancer is highest in the southern and western United States. This has long range implications as the population shifts to the sunbelt. It is particularly prevalent among fair skinned, light eyed people with skin that tans poorly and burns easily. Irish and Scottish people seem to be particularly susceptible, and Australia's increased incidence of skin cancers seems to parallel that of the United States.

What happens when sun strikes skin—when the first warm clear day comes and everyone heads for the outdoors to worship the sun and bask in the glow of good health? As radiation strikes the skin, some is thrown off the skin to the surface, making the skin feel warm to the touch; some is absorbed in the topmost layers of skin, and still more travels inward through deeper layers of skin, tissue and cells, which triggers the skin's defenses. Melanin is the skin's defense, the pigment deep within these cells that protects and filters the individual's skin, both from acute and chronic effects of exposure to the sun.

To Burn or to Tan? That Is the Question

Why don't you get much of a tan in Boston on a 30 degree day in February, even if the sun is shining brilliantly? Why do you get a wonderful suntan on that same day in February in the Bahamas, even if it is hazy and partly cloudy with a temperature of 70? Degree of tan is determined by both external and internal factors. The external factors which affect the degree of tanning or burning are: the wave lengths of the ultraviolet light, how far you are from the source, how long you are exposed, and what kind of surroundings you are in. For example, if you are in the sun from 10 o'clock until 2 o'clock, around water, snow, sand (reflective surfaces) or on a beach with no trees, the dose of radiation you are getting is very high. Naturally, in the Bahamas these factors are going to make you burn, but not much sunlight is reaching Boston in February.

The internal factors are: each individual's own skin color (the lighter the color, the more chance you will burn), previous exposures, thickness of the skin, amount of body hair, rare abnormal reactions, and the presence of antibiotics and other chemicals in your system.

The exposure to the sun stimulates the individual's output of pigment melanin. However, not everyone has the same number of pigment cells. The first category are Albinos, who have virtually no pigment cells. Second are redheads and other very fair skinned people who have very few pigment cells and never "tan." Included in this category are some slightly darker Caucasians that are able to tan slightly after burning first. A third and fourth category of Caucasians will tan with a moderate sunburn. The fifth category are olive skinned or Asian peoples who have more melanin, easily activated by the sun; they rarely burn and tan easily. The sixth category includes dark-skinned blacks who have heavily melanized pigment and rarely have difficulty absorbing or synthesizing the sun's ultraviolet rays.

The first step of sun tanning is immediate. Within a few minutes of exposure, the individual gets a nice reddish glow which lasts for about a half hour and fades shortly thereafter. This immediate reddish glow is followed by a delayed reddish glow which becomes maximum in 24 hours and subsides in the next few days. This healthy glow is really an illusion. The initial redness and slight swelling of the skin as it makes contact with the sun's rays tightens the face, thereby seeming to fade the wrinkles. Actually this "puffed up" effect is due to increased blood flow through the damaged superficial blood vessels of the skin. Those who have darker skin with more skin pigment are at an advantage here. Their skin thickens, scattering and absorbing the sun's rays more effectively. In the case of severe burns, the skin can blister and peel off after four to seven days. People in hot climates now use meters called Erythemameters to measure the exposure to the sun.

The second step is skin deep, the real suntan. It appears several days later, and lasts for a couple of months. It is the result of a synthesis of melanin to create new pigment. The efficiency of the body to do this work decreases with aging. Just like an often used rubber band, the skin gets thinner, loses its elasticity, and actually atrophies or withers from the process of expanding and contracting. This causes what sometimes is described romantically in men as a craggy, weather-beaten look; but in women it is a scourge of basic, garden-variety wrinkles.

Sunlight has a number of permanent effects on the different layers of the skin, and they all sustain damage over the years. The main target of ultraviolet radiation is DNA in the cells. When the skin is badly sunburned, some cells are killed off, and others are damaged. Some of the damaged cells can repair themselves completely, but for other cells, the DNA repair is incomplete. These are the cells that eventually become cancerous.

Skin cancer does not happen all at once. As we have said, the sun's damage is cumulative, and the changes in the skin go through an intermediate pre-cancerous stage. Called Actinic Keratoses, the skin forms hard, raised, grayish-colored patches that occur on areas of the body that have been exposed to years of sun. They should be differentiated from Seborrheic Keratoses which can occur all over the body and are not pre-cancerous.

Damage to the elastic tissue in the deeper layers of the skin is the cause of premature aging and wrinkling. The so-called Sailor's Skin or Farmer's Skin seen in Caucasians is the end result of prolonged exposure to sunlight. Recent research has shown that sunlight also impairs the functioning of the cells of the immune system which are located in the skin.

Other changes to the skin affect pigmentation. Sometimes, the skin actually loses its pigmentation and white areas will appear. The skin can also become hyper-pigmented, or darker in color. Some people develop liver spots as well.

These changes show up at the microscopic level. Lab experiments using ultraviolet-A light on chromosomes of cells have demonstrated that ultraviolet-A will "kink" the chromosomes if exposed to psoralen (a tar compound) even with short exposures. The human proof that ultraviolet-A causes cancer has been seen in patients treated with PUVA therapy (psoralen ultraviolet-A therapy).[9]

A Booth Full of Sun

Tanning booths, another popular "sunning" phenomenon have made an impact, particularly among the youth and young adults in our society. Getting a head start on your suntan, getting a tan in the privacy of a tanning booth, tanning all of those "hard to expose" areas — all have made these booths popular and profitable.

DID YOU KNOW THAT?

- There are approximately 18,000 free-standing tanning salons in the United States at present, just like fast food places.
- Between 6,000-7,000 health and fitness clubs in the United States have at least one tanning bed, and so do approximately 30,000 beauty salons.

Dr. G. Thomas Jenson, President of American Academy of Dermatology, is strongly urging the strict regulation of tanning facilities, which he feels is one of the most rapidly growing industries in the

Clinical Trials   **by Oidden**

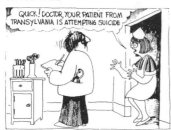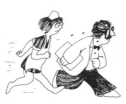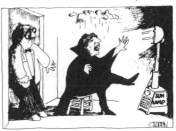

Reprinted with permission by Clinical Trials by Oidden, Medical Tribune, p.15, March 27, 1985

United States. This industry showed a 50 percent increase in 1987 alone and now, according to a Yellow Pages research group, there are 17,405 businesses listed. In the effort to educate society about the dangers of these tanning devices, the Food and Drug Administration (FDA) in cooperation with the American Academy of Dermatology has circulated a poster in 40,000 high schools around the United States. The FDA estimates that the sun lamps used in these salons give off about ten times more UV-A radiation than a session outdoors in the sun at high noon. The FDA regulations also allow tanning booths to use up to five percent UV-B light along with UV-A. Considering that most natural sunlight only contains one percent natural UV-B, the levels in artificial tanning booths are dangerously high.

These tanning salons are able to guarantee a "no-fail" tanning experience for this reason, and most of the people who use them think that they can get a good protective "base" of tan so they will not burn on a vacation. What a dreadful misunderstanding. Tanning is just the skin's reaction to injury from ultraviolet radiation.

The light from sunlamps is usually made of ultraviolet A rays. These rays are slightly longer than B rays, though the B rays are thought to be more damaging to the skin and more capable of causing genetic changes in epidermal and dermal cells that can ultimately lead to skin cancer. UV-A can also burn skin and corneas of the eyes differently than sunlight.

Skin cancer is the major side effect of using a sunlamp but it is not the only one. This artificial sunlight also suppresses the immune system. In one study, volunteers who attended 12 30-minute artificial tanning sessions in 14 days had lower scores on skin tests for immune capacity.

The FDA has certain requirements for safety when using sun lamps, and each sunlamp fixture must contain an FDA-approved warning. In addition, sun lamps must have a ten-minute or less timer, a manual switch, protective eye wear and a special base so lamps cannot be plugged into regular electric sockets. A recommended tanning schedule and suggested distance for placing the lamp from the user must also be included according to the FDA guidelines.

Sun Smarts and Sunscreens

It is neither healthy nor realistic to avoid the sun altogether. Sunlight makes us feel better and provides vitamin D for healthy bones. Tanning is the evidence of damage to skin. It is important to learn how to protect yourself from levels of exposure to the sun which are dangerous. This campaign has to start early in life. By age 20, the experts note, the typical American has received 80 percent of his or her lifetime exposure to skin damaging ultraviolet rays from sunlight. By adulthood, many children, particularly those who have fair skin and light eyes, who live in warm, sunny climates have had enough sun exposure to develop a skin cancer. Though the tan fades quickly after the summer, the ultraviolet damage has a cumulative effect that lasts a lifetime.

Commercially prepared sunscreen lotions and sunglasses, especially those that filter ultraviolet light, are essential for protection of skin and eyes. Regular use of a sunscreen with an SPF (Sun Protection Factor) of 15 for the first 18 years of a child's life reduces the lifetime incidence of skin cancer by 78 percent.[10]

Sunscreens are of two types: physical and chemical. Physical sunscreens are very effective in blocking ultraviolet radiation or sunlight from getting to the skin. They are usually salts of zinc and titanium, kaolin, iron oxide, etc., and they are available as white opaque pastes and creams. Since they are gritty and messy, lots of people prefer not to use them. Chemical sunscreens, which are colorless solutions, are more popular.

No one ingredient can offer full protection from UV-A and UV-B rays, so the best sunscreens combine several ingredients. Pick a product that is labelled "Broad Spectrum" to protect yourself. A popular ingredient in sunscreens is *PABA*, para-aminobenzoic acid, which works by scattering ultraviolet B. It has some drawbacks: it does not screen out UV-A; some people can be allergic to the alcohol or the fragrance or to the PABA itself; and it can cause acne in teenagers. Recently, according to testing done by the FDA, a nitrosamine was found in some sunscreens containing a PABA compound. A newer product with an SPF factor of 29 does not contain PABA, but uses another ingredient, octyl-methoxycinnamate.

Benzophenones (otherwise known as Oxybenzone, methoxybenzone, and sulfisobenzone) are good protection against UV-A rays, but less effective against UV-B. *Cinnamates* screen UV-B, but not as well as PABA. *Anthranilates* are moderately effective against both types of rays. Look for these ingredients on the labels.

Sunscreens are called suntan lotions but they do not promote tanning. In fact, they act to prevent it. A sunscreen low in PABA, such SPF 2, 4, or 6, is doing little to protect the skin beyond moisturizing it.

There are some problems with sunscreens. They need to be applied at least 30 minutes before going into the sun so that ingredients can penetrate the skin, and they should be re-applied after sweating or swimming, or routinely after two hours in the sun. Oil based products stay on better through swimming and perspiring, and people who want the most effective protection should use two different sunscreens—one for reflecting and the other for absorbing the sun's rays. There has also been new evidence raising concerns about the chemical safety of some sunscreens.

Clear liquids and lotions that do not stain are the most desirable, but there are reflector sunscreens, usually thick and opaque with a high degree of zinc oxide that blocks out sun for specific areas such as the nose, lips, and cheeks. A California company produced this product in a series of fluorescent colors which have been popular among teenagers at the beach. Whether liquid, lotion or cream, sunbathers need to make certain that they have covered all of the areas of exposed skin.

Dr. William Hanke, Assistant Professor of Dermatology at the Indiana State Medical Center, has recommended some important precautions:[11]

- At the beginning of summer, start with sun exposure for 15 minutes on the first day, and not more than 30 minutes for a few subsequent days.

- You should limit outdoor activities between 11 a.m. and 2 p.m. whether it is sunny or cloudy.

- If you are near sand, snow, concrete or water, you are at a higher risk for sunburn because of the increased reflection of ultraviolet light.

- Wear wide-brimmed hats, like sombreros, cotton shirts with long sleeves, cotton long-legged pants and goggles.

- Sun screens should be applied on lips, ears, nose and other exposed areas.

- Always reapply the sunscreen after swimming or bathing.

The Skin Cancer Foundation releases a list of sunscreens it feels "aid in the prevention of sun induced damage to the skin." To receive their current list, call (212) 725-5176, or write: The Skin Cancer Foundation, 245 Fifth Avenue, Suite 2402, New York, NY 10016.

RADON GAS: THE PARADOXICAL POLLUTANT

Air and water pollution and toxic substances are all negative offshoots of man-made "progress". As if there were not enough problems to worry about from these conventional pollutants, now there is radon. EPA estimates radon exposure is responsible for up to 20,000 lung cancers in the United States annually.[12]

Tasteless, odorless, and invisible, radon is a breakdown product of uranium as it turns into non-radioactive lead and a natural part of our universe. Low level radioactive gases such as radon are ubiquitous, and like low level exposure to the sun, create no health problems. Underground, the gas can travel for miles through soil and water, rising to the earth's surface through porous rocks and faults. Outdoors the gas is not a health hazard for it is absorbed quickly into the atmosphere. But in confined, tightly sealed spaces where there is little ventilation, like our energy-efficient homes and our temperature controlled, electronically heated and air-cooled buildings, watch out! Radon gas can build up to a deadly concentration.

There are three ways that radioactive radon gas can enter buildings: transported with soil through cracks and openings in the foundation; emanating from earth-derived building materials, sump pumps, exposed dirt floors in basements, cracks or gaps in concrete foundations, concrete block or cinder block walls; and finally, transported through water and natural gas.

Through one of these pathways, radon entered the Boyertown, Pennsylvania, home of Diane and Stanley Watras in 1985. For Watras, an engineer for Bechtel, radon was as imperceptible as breathing. He could not understand why he was setting off the radiation monitors at the Limerick nuclear power plant where he worked near Boyertown, Pennsylvania. Strangely, he was setting off the monitors in the mornings when he arrived at work, rather than in the evenings when he left. There were some other facts about radon that Watras did not understand. He didn't know that his house was situated in the region geologists call the Reading Prong, stretching from Reading, Pennsylvania, to New Jersey and New York state, and full of "Radon Hot Spots." These are areas with uranium decay in large deposits of shale, granite and phosphate.

Watras was not destined to remain naive much longer. He asked the plant's owner, The Philadelphia Electric Company, to check radiation levels in his home. The results of the air samples came as a total shock. For one year, Watras and his wife had been living in a home in which

53

the air was saturated with enough radioactivity to equal exposure to 455,000 chest X-rays!

The newly constructed well-insulated home that the Watrases had bought was harboring the highest concentration of radon ever found in the United States. In this one year of exposure, the Watrases had increased their risk of contacting lung cancer over the course of their lifetimes by 14 percent.

The Environmental Resources Department of the State of Pennsylvania was just as shocked and began testing other houses in the immediate area around Boyertown. The results after five months of air sampling? The Watras' house was no fluke; over forty percent of the homes in the surrounding area had unacceptably high concentrations of radon gas.

The Watras' house was not at fault. If anything, it was constructed too well—too tightly sealed and too well-insulated to vent the dangerous concentration of radioactive gas and its by-products. Even the location could not be blamed, for concentrations of radon can vary dramatically from neighborhood to neighborhood, house to house.

Interest and concern in the radon problem snowballed. In 1986, within a year of the Watras' discovery, the Environmental Protection Agency issued ominous warnings that radon and its radioactive decay products (called "daughters") posed a public health threat of sweeping proportions to as many as eight million American homes and could be responsible for up to 20,000 lung cancer deaths in the United States each year.

The menace from radon comes from its unique properties as well as it commonplace ones. Radon is present in such common building materials as brick and concrete, rocks such as granite and shale, and even soil. Unlike the other elements in the cascade from uranium to lead which are stable and tend to stay locked up in the minerals where they form, radon drifts and moves through rocks and soil unattached to other chemical elements. Some radon enters the air this way before it decays into its "daughter" products, but these products are the most destructive to human lung tissue.

A Little Bit of Alpha Goes a Very Long Way

Some of the daughter products of radon emit alpha particles, depositing their load in small sections of tissue—but what a load: *alpha particles have the potential to inflict 10 to 20 times the biological damage to tissue as electrons or X-rays of similar energy.* Generally, the DNA in the nucleus of these cells in the human is the site of damage from radon daughters, and damage to the DNA can cause the cell to grow uncontrollably—in other words, the beginnings of a cancer cell.

Radiation can also disrupt enough chemical bonds of a chromosome to break it into fragments, resulting in "mutation." This process does not happen all at once. Scientists first understood the dangers of radon as a carcinogenic agent back in 1900 when it was noted that uranium miners were subject to unusually high rates of lung cancer, occurring after a latency period of about 20 years between exposure and onset.

What is new about radon is the human factor. Changes in life styles and working habits in our post-industrial high-tech society means that the general population in the United States spends about 80 percent of its time indoors. With increased attention to energy conservation, "indoors" often implies tightly sealed buildings that may not be well-ventilated. The problem is not limited to occupations such as uranium mining, or to houses built with left-over uranium tailings from the foundations of nearby-by mines—the situation in Grand Junction, Colorado, in the 1950s, or in the New Jersey cities of Montclair and Vernon.

Especially since the media coverage of the Watrases' experiences in 1984-85, the general population has been made aware of the potential dangers of this invisible indoor pollutant in everyday settings and situations. This consciousness-raising happened quickly. Within a few months of the discovery of the Watrases' bad fortune, governmental agencies such as the EPA began attempting to respond to the challenge. EPA officials believe radon could be everywhere. No one knows just how many radon tainted sites there are throughout the United States and how many homes might be harboring unsafe concentrations of the radioactive gas. In conjunction with state health departments, the EPA has developed a survey method for testing patterns of radon contamination and has estimated that ten percent of the homes in the United States have radon concentrations above four picocuries. In 1986, the EPA established federal standards for levels at which radon indoors should be considered a serious risk and made recommendations for dealing with it.

The National Council on Radiation Protection and Measurements has set four picocuries (radiation intensity) per liter of air as the upper limit of safe levels for long term human exposure, based on epidemiological studies of uranium workers. The presence of one picocurie is about average for most homes in the United States, and ten or more is considered dangerous enough to require immediate attention. Dr. Jerome Marmorstein at the University of Southern California assesses the lifetime risk of death from lung cancer from average radon exposure in the United States is 0.4 percent.[13]

Certain geographical areas are known to have greater amounts of radon than others. Besides the Reading Prong of Pennsylvania, New

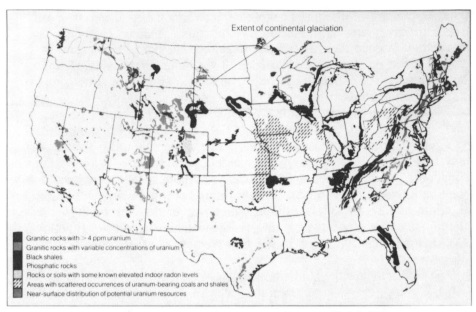

Extent of continental glaciation

Granitic rocks with > 4 ppm uranium
Granitic rocks with variable concentrations of uranium
Black shales
Phosphatic rocks
Rocks or soils with some known elevated indoor radon levels
Areas with scattered occurrences of uranium-bearing coals and shales
Near-surface distribution of potential uranium resources

Reprinted with permission from The Journal of Respiratory Disease, P. 75, July 1989

Areas with potentially high indoor radon levels are represented by the shaded regions on this map; however, areas outside these regions are not free of risk from high indoor radon levels. Potential radon levels are based solely on the uranium content of rocks near the surface (see legend). The extent of continental glaciation indicates where glacial material may cover bedrock; soil characteristics north of this line may affect radon levels more than underlying rock. This map cannot be used to predict high radon levels in specific localities or to identify levels in individual homes, since local variations, including soil permeability and housing characteristics strongly affect indoor radon levels and regional predictions.

U.S. Environmental Agency Map, Washington, D.C. Based on geological reports, modified National Uranium Resource Evaluation data, and some indoor radon data, August 1987. No information available on Alaska and Hawaii.

York, and New Jersey, there are high concentrations of uranium in Maine, New Hampshire, central Florida, Idaho, Montana, the Carolinas, Georgia, Texas, California, and Washington state. In fact, the agency has established its existence in 30 states, although concentrations vary.

What Can You Do?

For the Watrases, it took 32,000 dollars to make their radon-tainted home habitable again, an expense which was paid for by Stanley's company. Many of Watrases' neighbors, however, faced having to make a painful value decision; they have had to choose whether to pay for the expensive clean-up themselves, live with the increased cancer risks, or simply move out and jeopardize their most important possession and investment.

Government involvement is another question. At what level of risk should the government step in, offering subsidies to the needy for corrective clean-ups? What kinds of legislation can governments support?

Individual homeowners can test their own homes for radon using two types of available do-it-yourself kits. A quick test which takes about one week consists of a sealed canister containing activated charcoal. The canister is unsealed and placed in the lowest living area of the home. At the end of the monitoring period, the canister is re-sealed and sent to the manufacturer for an analysis, which consists of counting the radioactive emissions produced by radon decay products. This type of test runs 12-15 dollars. Information on do-it-yourself Radon testing kits can be obtained from:

> Air Check 1-800-247-2435
> Radon Project 1-412-687-3393

Another test, which takes 90 days, is called an "alpha track" test because it measures tracks made in a special plastic by the radioactive decay particles. Like the charcoal canisters, the alpha-track capsules are placed in a draft-free area and left alone for the duration of the test. They are more accurate than the shorter-term test because they are less susceptible to daily variations caused by weather or other factors. This test costs around 50 dollars. Information on this type of test can be obtained by calling:

> Rad Track 1-800-528-8327

Homeowners who want to know whether radon is leaking into their home should place a test capsule in the basement. Those who want to know personal exposure levels should choose the least frequently used living area.

The range of content of radioactive substances in common building materials varies greatly, so methods for radon reduction depend on the specific situation, and the level of radiation.

The easiest solution to a higher than normal radon count is simply to increase air exchange by opening windows and using fans. The tradeoff—higher energy and fuel bills. Another solution for sealing concrete and small leaks in basements is to use a good quality paint.

Water supplies in the household are another major source of radon. Rural homeowners are at a disadvantage here for water from drilled wells appears to have higher concentrations of radon than that of lakes and city reservoirs.

Inexpensive changes in building construction practices can make big improvements for the future. Site selection should be carefully checked, and placing drain pipes outside the house's footings rather than within, can eliminate a major conduit for radon gas.

For existing property, a variety of measures must be applied. Researchers have found that some houses draw radon gas up from the ground almost as chimneys do, resulting from differences in air pressure between the inside of a radon-tainted house and the ground below it. If ventilation is not adequate, the radon gas level builds up. In these cases, air-to-air heat exchangers are another solution. These consist of a core, two fans, and two filters, all mounted in an insulated case. One fan brings outdoor air in through the core and into the house. As the air passes through the core, heat is transferred across a thin partition from the warmer to the cooler airstream. Thus, in the winter the supply air is warmed before entering the house, and the exhaust air is cooled before leaving the house. The reverse process can keep the heat outside over the summer. Most residential models of heat exchangers can be connected to existing duct work. Federal and state agencies are experimenting with ways to reduce the flow of radon into buildings or to dissipate it quickly once it is inside.

Only by being informed about the potential dangers to one's own home and future health can the individual make wise choices. The EPA has recommended that all homes in the United States be tested for Radon. Presumably about 10-15 percent of the homes are estimated to have radon levels above EPA's "action level" of four picocuries per litre. The EPA estimates the highest levels of radon are in Minnesota and North Dakota.

More information about Radon Gas may be obtained from your local health department, or by writing to:

S.M. Woods
Consumer Information Center
Pueblo, Colorado, 81009
(Request Item No. 136R)

OR

Environmental Protection Agency
401 M Street S.W.
Suite 200, North East Mall
Washington, D.C. 20460
(202) 475-9605

For further reading on radon, I would suggest the book *Radon: The Invisible Threat* by Michael Lafavore.[14]

RADIATION IN THE HOME: MICROWAVE, TELEVISION AND HOME COMPUTERS

Microwave ovens use high levels of microwave radiation to cook food by adding energy to it. Metal casings and screens in the oven should stop the radiation from settling into the food. The only problems here can come from leakage, especially around the door seals. Leakage from microwaves are suspected of causing cancer of the red blood cells, called polycythemia. Three things to remember: keep door seals clean, never run the oven while empty, and discourage young children from standing too close and peering into the screen to "see what's cooking."

Picture tubes in television sets work by stopping or slowing high speed electrons, and this produces X-rays. Most, but not all, tubes in radios, TV sets and computer display terminals operate at low voltages which limit the power of the X-rays produced so that they are contained by the glass tube. The only significant problems here can come from older TV sets, particularly color TV sets built before January 15, 1970, when the industry had less stringent X-ray emission standards.

There are currently 15 million video display terminals (VDTs) being used in the United States; the number is expected to increase to 100 million by the year 2000.[15] Color display terminals give off slightly more radiation than black-and-white ones, but radiation leakage should not be a problem in units that are working properly.

Office video display terminals present a more concentrated problem. Ten to fourteen million office workers in the United States and Canada sit in front of a video display terminal for long hours each day, and these numbers are growing rapidly as more firms and homes "computerize." At present there are no large-scale epidemiological studies to correlate health problems with long hours of exposure to video display terminals. Like TV sets, there should be no serious leakage problems if these terminals are working properly. There have been isolated clusters of complaints such as stress, cataracts, and even increased incidence of birth defects and miscarriages, but it is too soon to have convincing data.

It is important to keep in mind that these video display terminals do emit a wide range of radiation, though in low levels, and could produce health problems in combination with other elements.

ELECTRICAL AND MAGNETIC FIELDS

There are over 300,000 miles of alternating current transmission lines that are stretched across the United States. There is a growing suspicion that the magnetic fields that are created around the transformers on these power lines are related to childhood cancer. It has been seen that children living in homes close to power lines have a higher rate of cancer, a finding supported by a recent study done in Denver, Colorado.[16] Dr. David Carpenter of the New York State Health Department believes that, in general, people working in "electrical" occupations such as radar maintenance workers have higher rates of leukemia, lymphoma and brain tumors.[17]

A study was done in 1982 in Washington state on workers in occupations with exposure to electrical and magnetic fields in the years from 1950-1979, showing that they had increased risk of death due to leukemia. A similar trend has been seen in amateur radio operators according to Dr. Wilham of Washington State Department of Social and Health Services.[18]

MEDICAL AND DENTAL RADIATION

X-rays were first discovered by Roentgen in 1895 and were quickly adopted by the medical profession to diagnose all kinds of medical ills. They revolutionized the diagnosis and treatment of many illnesses. X-rays are a very useful and widely used diagnostic and therapeutic modality.

DID YOU KNOW THAT?

- Each year approximately 160 million Americans undergo 250 million diagnostic X-ray exams.

- Of these, about 45 million Americans have a routine X-ray each year for reasons of occupation, admission to hospital, government service, college or other institution.

- About 50 percent of all X-ray exams involve the chest, at an annual cost of two billion dollars? Many of these exams are performed on asymptomatic subjects.

- One percent of all cases of leukemia and 0.7 percent of all cases of breast cancer that occur annually in the United States can be attributed to lifetime exposure to diagnostic radiation.

- Between 50-60 percent of all exposure to radiation in the United States population comes from medical or dental X-rays, the other half coming mostly from natural background sources.[19]

Diagnostic X-rays

How dangerous are medical X-rays? When does the diagnostic tool pose as great a risk as the disease? Again, like considering the potential dangers of radon, the individual has to make a value judgment and weigh the benefits as well as the risks.

X-ray, since its discovery, has been one of medicine's most remarkable tools. It penetrates deep into the recesses of the body where light cannot pass and where physical examination would be impossible. The benefits in diagnosing everything from kidney stones, tumors, fractures to tooth decay are obvious. But X-ray can be used indiscriminately, and it can expose the individual to radiation unnecessarily. Some offshoots of X-ray, equally hazardous, include fluoroscopy (continuous X-ray) and CAT scans (computer controlled X-ray system which can take cross-sectional views of internal organs). This risk versus benefit should be evaluated each time X-rays are used for diagnosis of a disease. We know that many people take great risks all the time, risks which range from bull fighting, skydiving, mountain climbing and flying an airplane to crossing a street carelessly. In short, even though there is a small risk of cancer from an X-ray diagnosis, it should be done if it is necessary for making a diagnosis.

Generally the average dose of radiation received by humans is 0.17 rad/year, from natural and man-made radiation sources. (A milliard is 1/1,000 of a rad). X-ray exams can fall into High, Medium, or Low dose categories:

HIGH DOSE: (more than 125 mrads per average exam) Mammography, Upper Gastrointestinal, Thoracic spine, Lower Gastrointestinal, Lumbosacral spine and CAT Scans.

MEDIUM DOSE: (25-125 mrads per average exam) Intravenous pyelogram, Cervical spine, Cholecystography, KUB and Skull.

LOW DOSE: (less than 25 mrads per average exam) Chest, Hip Shoulder, Extremities and Dental.

There are *250 million* radiological procedures performed each year in the United States, and the average exposure to an individual is 0.08 rad in the bone marrow. The estimated cancer risk from most diagnostic X-ray procedures is one case per million procedures per year. The risk of cancer is much higher if the exposures are high. Patients who had repeated fluoroscopy suffer from a higher incidence of breast cancer, and patients exposed to thorotrast (a highly radioactive material) for diagnosis of liver disease now suffer from high rates of liver cancer.

MAXIMUM PERMISSIBLE DOSE OF X-RAYS PER YEAR	
Whole Body, Eye, Blood forming Organs	5 rem
Skin	15 rem
Hands	75 rem
Other Organs (Thyroid)	15 rem
Pregnant Women (Total During Gestation)	0.5 rem

Goodbye Routine X-rays

Four X-ray procedures have raised controversy because of their widespread use, largely on asymptomatic patients in mass screening programs. They are: routine chest X-ray to detect tuberculosis and cancer; mammography to detect possible breast cancer; scoliosis X-ray for school children to detect deformity in the spine; and finally, dental X-rays. Each presents an example of a productive, and an unproductive screening program. First, let us consider mammography.

Mammography

In the United States today, about 70,000 new cases of breast cancer are diagnosed annually and about 38,000 women die of the disease. The breast and thyroid, along with bone marrow, are three areas that are highly sensitive to the effects of ionizing radiation. Dr. Nancy A. Finnerty of the M.D. Anderson Hospital in Houston believes that the breasts are most sensitive to the carcinogenic effect of radiation during the second decade of life up to age thirty, the period of greatest breast development. Yet, early detection is an important factor in breast cancer cure rates, so much so that mammography screening programs, practiced over a 30 year period, could reduce the number of deaths due to breast cancer each year by one third. But at what price?

Mammography techniques have improved over the past ten years, exposing women to much lower doses of radiation. In conjunction with

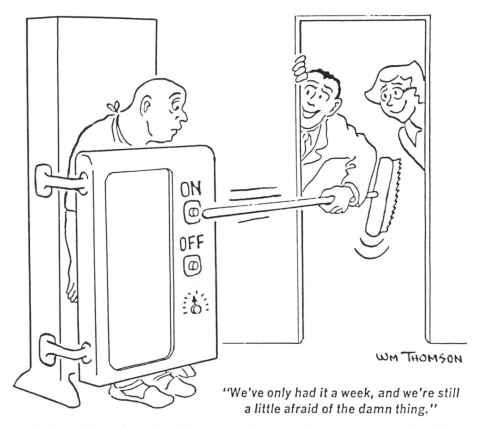

*"We've only had it a week, and we're still
a little afraid of the damn thing."*

Reprinted with permission from Moor Cartoon Classics, Medical Economics Co., p.97, 1973

physical exams, mammography has been found to be highly effective in early detection of breast cancer. A study was done by the Health Insurance Plan of New York in 1960 for screening for breast cancer. The screen group was given a physical exam and a mammogram, while the control group only received routine medical care. In the screen group women 50 and over showed a 25-30 percent reduction in deaths after ten to 14 years. Studies done by the National Cancer Institute and the American Cancer Society Breast Cancer Detection and Demonstration Project (1973-90) involved over 275,000 women who had physical exams and mammograms. More than 41 percent of the cancers were detected early with the mammogram—most in early stages, offering a high possibility of cure.[20]

The current recommendations follow: for women without symptoms, 40 to 49-year-olds should have a yearly physical exam and a mammogram every one to two years, depending upon risk factors; for women aged 50 or over, they should have a yearly physical exam and mammogram. All symptomatic women of any age should rely on advice given by their physician.

Chest X-rays

Fifty two million chest X-rays were done in United States hospitals in 1980, making chest X-rays the most frequently used procedure in the United States. Sixty percent of these chest X-rays were routine, costing 1.5 billion dollars.[21] Chest X-ray is another widely practiced procedure performed on healthy, asymptomatic people. For many occupations— school teachers, nurses and food handlers—as well as every patient admitted into a nursing home or hospital, yearly X-rays are a common practice. However, many experts feel the X-ray has outlived its usefulness as a mass screening diagnostic tool.

A panel of physicians representing the specialties of radiology, thoracic medicine, family practice, epidemiology and occupational medicine was formed by the Food and Drug Administration's National Center for Devices and Radiological Health (NCDRH) to study this issue. After extensive evaluation, this chest X-ray panel concluded that the yield of unsuspected heart disease, lung cancer and tuberculosis found in routine screening chest X-rays unaccompanied by history, physical exams or specific diagnostic testing has been shown to be of insufficient clinical value to justify the monetary cost, added radiation exposure, and inconvenience of the exam. Their recommendations follow:

- Discontinue all routine screening exams of unselected populations unless a significant yield can be shown;
- All routine prenatal chest X-ray screening exams for detection of unsuspected disease should be discontinued;
- Routine chest X-rays should not be required solely because of hospital admission;
- Mandated chest X-ray exams because of employment, institutional admission, or of TB follow-up patients are shown to be of insufficient clinical value to continue their use;
- Routine non-selective chest X-ray exams related to job, re-employment or annual employment should be discontinued.

The American College of Radiology, The American Academy of Family Physicians, The American College of Obstetricians and Gynecologists, The American Thoracic Society, and the American College of Occupational Medicine have all endorsed the Chest X-ray Panel's conclusions.

In 1980 the United States Surgeon General announced the discontinuation of routine chest X-ray exams for Public Health Service employees, or about 32,000 X-ray exams each year—amounting to a saving of four million dollars annually, and asked other Federal agencies to review their position on this issue.

A problem is that many patients do not feel that a physical examination is complete unless they have had an X-ray. An X-ray shows definitively that everything is in order. Also, as part of our litigious age and the propensity for malpractice suits, many physicians feel compelled to practice "defensive medicine" and document every diagnosis. What better way than the concrete evidence of an X-ray? One of the top radiation physicists today, Dr. John W. Gofman, writes that, in a way, lawyers are a cause of cancer.[22]

Scoliosis

Another recent FDA concern is the increased number of spinal X-rays in United States' public schools for screening for scoliosis. Two-thirds of those referred for follow-up X-rays for scoliosis are females.[23] A "follow-up" usually means one or more radiographs on each visit, made as often as every three months until the patient reaches skeletal maturity.

Pre-adolescent and adolescent girls with developing breasts are particularly sensitive to the carcinogenic effects of radiation, and special care must be taken to use fast X-ray film/screen techniques for minimum exposure, shields over the breast, and posteroanterior rather than anteroposterior projection. Fortunately, a recent development of a new imaging system cuts down radiation exposure to the body to negligible levels by a system called the Integrated Shape Imaging System (ISIS).

Dental X-rays

Dental X-rays are not without risk, and X-ray equipment varies dramatically from one dentist to the next. In 1982, radiation expert J.W. Gofman calculated the cancer risk for different age groups based on having five dental X-ray films taken per year. This was the American average number of X-rays taken per dental visit in 1972. Among those who had five films per year from age seven to age 45, Dr. Gofman found the risk for leukemia, mouth and throat cancer, and brain cancer to be one in every 251 males, one out of every 514 females, a risk level much higher than for the general population.

The FDA, in their concern about the general public's exposure to unnecessary X-rays, has released guidelines about use of dental X-rays. These guidelines have been developed after consulting with several professional dental organizations. They have stressed that asymptomatic patients should have dental X-rays only after a thorough history and physical examination has been done.

Early Exposure to X-rays

In the mid-1930s to mid-1950s, X-ray was considered to be a biomedical miracle, a diagnostic tool and even a cure for just about everything. Because there were no antibiotics available, patients, particularly children, were often treated with X-ray for such common-place medical problems as whooping cough, ringworm in the scalp, enlarged tonsils, and enlarged glands in the neck, etc. Upon reaching adulthood, these infants and children were found to have a much higher incidence of thyroid cancer, a type of cancer which can be a health concern for a particularly long period of time, up to 35 years after initial exposure.

A famous long-term study done by Dr. Murray J. Favus and his associates at the Michael Reese Hospital in Chicago followed over 1,000 people that received 700-900 rads to the head and neck area when they were children.[24] Surgery was done on 182 of these control patients as adults, and thyroid cancer was detected in 60 of these, which is over five percent of the total patients. The cancers detected were of the skin, thyroid and parotid glands. One way to reduce the risk of thyroid cancer is to use lead collars to cover the thyroid in patients who are getting radiation to the head and neck areas.[25]

Pregnancy and X-rays

X-rays during pregnancy and fetal X-rays are another head start on X-ray exposure, and were, again, a common procedure in the 1930s and 1940s in many obstetrical practices. In a survey done in Oxford, England, Drs. Alice Stewart and J. F. Bithell, British researchers, published findings that stated that unborn fetuses with a history of radiation exposure doubled the risk of a variety of childhood cancers and leukemias by age ten.[26] A study done by Dr. Brian MacMahon, a Harvard researcher in the United States, also showed an increased risk of cancer in these children who had X-ray exposure when their mothers were pregnant.[27] Recent research by Dr. E. Harvey and associates of the National Cancer Institute showed that an exposure to one to four rads raised the cancer risk in children by 40-50 percent and raised the risk even higher in twins.[28]

Radiation as a Cure

X-rays have been used since their discovery to treat both cancer and non-cancerous conditions like rheumatoid arthritis, tuberculosis, and arthritis in the spine as well as many head and neck conditions. All these patients have been found to be at high risk for cancer, depending upon the dose of and the area of the body exposed to radiation.

There are approximately *two million* Americans alive today who have been cured of cancer. About 50 percent of them owe their lives to the use of radiation as therapy. In the Western world, where cancer affects one out of three persons and will kill one out of four people, half of these patients will be treated with radiation at some point. In addition, radiotherapy is still used for benign conditions in about five percent. So overall, ten percent of the Western population will be treated with radiation therapy sometime during their lifetime.[29]

Radiation treatment works on cancer cells by making cells incapable of reproduction, and thereby destroying them. The problem is that it is not always so easy to hit the apple and miss William Tell. There is always some spill-over of radiation to the normal surrounding tissues. Therefore, X-ray doses must be calculated very carefully and aimed accurately at the cancerous area.

Radiation treatments are administered either by external treatment or with a radiation source placed in the patient's body. External treatments can be delivered in two manners: as gamma rays (X-rays) or as electron beams. The X-rays vary in voltage increasing up to megavoltage (over one million volts) depending upon how deep the tumor is located. The latest equipment, linear accelerators, can operate at up to eight million volts and reach even the deepest of tumors.

Internal radiation therapy, brachytherapy, is the implantation of sealed radio-nuclides directly to the cancerous part of the body. This is another innovative use of therapeutic radiation and is used successfully in cervical cancers and cancers of the prostate, head, and tongue. Radioactive Iodine 131 is used in the treatment of thyroid cancer and radioactive phosphorus [P-32] is used for red blood cell cancer called Polycythemia vera.

There are hazards associated with the use of radiation treatments. The most important of these is the second cancer caused by radiation treatment of the first. The risk appears to be *ten times greater* for both children and adults as compared to the general population. A very important study in this area was done by the Late Effect Study Group which found a higher incidence of leukemia, soft tissue, thyroid and breast cancers, in children treated for cancers with chemotherapy and radiation.[30]

NUCLEAR POWER

The atomic age is here to stay. Radium was first discovered by Madam Marie Curie in 1898, and other radioactive materials were discovered later. These were quickly put into commercial use. The first use of radioactive materials was painting of luminous watch dials in the luminizing industry. This was done by hand, and the paint brush was frequently pointed by workers with their lips before painting the dials. Consequently, the radioactive paint found entry into the body. Nine-hundred workers in New Jersey and Connecticut were exposed to radiation between 1917 and 1924, and many suffered from bone cancer.

Another radioactive material, thorotrast (containing Thorium) was used as a diagnostic agent in 1940-50. Some of these patients are now at high risk for lung cancer and leukemia.

During the Second World War, research of atomic materials produced the atomic bomb. The workers involved in manufacturing these bombs have an increased risk of cancer. Also at higher risk for cancers such as leukemia and thyroid cancer are the participants in the nuclear tests and residents of communities where the bombs were tested—the Marshall Islands, Bikini Islands, and the southwestern United States.

Finally, the era of peaceful uses of nuclear energy arrived when the USSR built the first nuclear power plant for generating electricity. Nuclear power later became quite popular in Europe and in the United States, and now many countries have nuclear power plants. Accidents involving these plants have happened. There was a movie released in the late 70s called "China Syndrome," which was sort of a doomsday prediction about what can happen to these nuclear power plants that are so close to where we live; the Three Mile Island accident happened shortly after the release of the film. The worst accident of all time occurred in 1986 in Chernobyl, the USSR. Protests were held world-wide about the delayed and inadequate Soviet response to the accident and general mismanagement of the industry.

Chernobyl

In April, 1986, one of the reactors at Chernobyl in the southwest Soviet Union ripped open and blew its top—spilling all its smoke and radioactive gases into the environment. There was a huge fallout of atomic materials into the air, soil and the neighboring Kiev River. Even cattle feed and cattle were polluted with radioactivity. The plume of radioactive gases spread into northern Europe, Ireland, and as far as the United States. The main component of these gases is radioactive iodine which has a half life of eight days, which means that it loses half of its radioactivity after eight days. Current estimates are that it cost four billion dollars to clean up and contain the damaged reactor. Up to 75,000 people have been exposed and will suffer from cancer of the thyroid, breast, lungs and leukemia over the next 100 years. It will take many, many years to clean up all of this radioactivity.

The remedy in a situation like this is to take stable iodine to saturate the thyroid gland so that it won't pick up radioactivity. This was done during the Chernobyl nuclear accident.

The workers that are at highest risk are temporary workers called "jumpers" because they are assigned high risk repair jobs within the nuclear reactors. However, risk of exposure to nuclear materials affects everyone, not just the workers in the plants.

LOW LEVEL RADIOACTIVE WASTE (LLRW) — NOT IN *MY* BACK YARD

The proper disposal of low-level radioactive waste is a problem with far-reaching consequences. (The term "low-level radioactive waste" is actually a misnomer, as radioactive waste remains radioactive for hundreds and thousands of years.) In 1985 nearly three million cubic feet of LLRW were generated in the United States by utilities, industries, hospitals, universities and pharmaceuticals. According to Jeff Smiley, Manager of the Department of Energy's Civilian Radioactive Waste Program, 64 percent of LLRW comes from the utility companies and consists of contaminated booties and mittens worn in the contaminated area, as well as sludge filters and contaminated metal parts of the reactors. Twenty-eight percent of the LLRW comes from pharmaceutical industry, six percent from labs in the universities and hospitals and two percent from the Navy.[31]

Disposal of this waste has always been a problem. In the 1950s, the waste was generally dumped into the sea or buried at federal sites. But many of these old sites are not used anymore. There are three new sites in Beatty, Nevada; Barnwell, South Carolina; and Hanford, Washington. These three states are dissatisfied with the arrangement, and the federal government has plans to make eight regional compacts throughout the country. It has become clear, however, that no one wants this dangerous waste in their backyard.

CHAPTER FOUR NOTES

1. Philip Hilts, *New York Times*, (Dec. 1989)
2. Skin Cancer Foundation, *Primary Care and Cancer,* (May 1990)
3. G.M. Findlay, *Lancet*, (1928)
4. Harold P. Rusch, et. al., *Archives of Pathology*, (1941)

5. Andrew Glass and Robert Hoover, *Journal of the American Medical Association*, (Oct. 20, 1989)

6. Skin Cancer Foundation, *Primary Care and Cancer*, (May 1990)

7. *Ibid.*

8. A. Sober and T.J. Fitzpatrick, "Sunlight and Skin Cancer, Editorial," *New England Journal of Medicine*, (Sept. 1985)

9. American Medical Association's Council of Scientific Affairs, *Journal of the American Medical Association*, (July 21, 1989)

10. *Archives of Dermatology*, 122: (1986)

11. William Hanke, "Eleven Ways to Protect Yourself from the Sun," *Your Patient and Cancer*, (July 1983)

12. *Journal of the American Medical Association*, (Nov. 1989)

13. Jerome Marmorstein, *Medical Tribune*, (Dec. 1988)

14. Michael Lafavore, *Radon: The Invisible Threat*, (Rodale Press, 1987)

15. Council on Scientific Affairs Report, *Journal of the American Medical Association*, (March 1987)

16. Robert S. Banks, *Health and Environment Digest*, (March 1988)

17. David Carpenter, *Health and Environment Digest*, (March 1988)

18. Wilham, *American Journal of Epidemiology*, (1987)

19. John Boise, Jr., "The Dangers of X Rays — Real or Apparent?" *New England Journal of Medicine*, (Sept. 1986)

20. Kopans, *New England Journal of Medicine*, (April 4, 1984)

21. Hubbell, *New England Journal of Medicine*, (Jan. 1985)

22. John W. Gofman, *Radiation and Human Health*, (Sierra Club Books, 1981)

23. "Protecting the Breast During Scoliosis Radiography," FDA, *Drug Bulletin*, (April 1985)

24. Murray J. Favus, et.al., *New England Journal of Medicine*, (May 1976)

25. Herbert Goldschmidt, *Archives of Dermatology*, (May 1983)

26. Alice Stewart and J. F. Bithell, *British Journal of Cancer*, (1975)

27. Brian MacMahon, "Prenatal X Ray Exposure and Childhood Cancer in Twins," *Journal of National Cancer Institute*, Vol. 29 (May 1982)

28. Elizabeth Harvey, et. al., "Prenatal X Ray Exposure and Childhood Cancer in Twins," *New England Journal of Medicine*, (Feb. 1985)

29. Brian O'Sullivan and Simon B. Sutcliffe, "The Toxicity of Radiotherapy," *Clinics in Oncology*, (Nov. 1985)

30. *Ibid.*

31. *Environmental Action*, Jan. 1986

CHAPTER FIVE

CHEMICALS: AT HOME AND IN THE WORK PLACE

Both the public and scientific community have long been concerned about exposure to the hazardous and carcinogenic chemicals in the home and workplace. The first account of cancer related to occupation was in 1774; the English physician Percival Pott noticed higher rates for cancer in chimney sweepers. Since then a large body of scientific evidence has been accumulated, showing that up to 40 percent of all cancers are caused by exposure to chemical pollution in air, water, food and soil— both at home and at work.

The Health and Human Services National Toxicology Program estimates that there are about 60,000 chemicals in the United States presently, and 700-1,000 new commercial chemicals are introduced every year.[1] Most of these chemicals have never been tested and are not regulated. Only seven industrial processes are regulated. Only 23 chemicals are listed as definite human carcinogens, while 61 are designated as probable human carcinogens. According to Dr. Marie Swanson of the Michigan Cancer Foundation in Detroit, by 1986, 39 chemicals in the workplace were regulated as human carcinogens by Occupational Safety and Health Administration (OSHA).

In the latter half of the 20th century there has been unprecedented growth in the petrochemical industry. Dr. Samuel Epstein of the

University of Illinois School of Public Health writes that the production of synthetic organic chemicals has exploded in the United States; it was one billion pounds in 1935, 30 billion pounds in 1950, and 300 billion pounds in 1975 alone.[2] Studies of cancer rates have shown parallel patterns of increase. Natural gas and crude oil is distilled further to make products as diverse as fuel for our automobiles, plastics, solvents, dyes, and pesticides.

All workers in the chemical industry and residents of communities where the plants are located are exposed to carcinogens daily. A number of studies have been done on oil refinery workers, petrochemical workers, chemists and researchers who are exposed to these chemicals, showing higher than average incidence of skin cancer, lung cancer, brain tumors, lymphomas, and leukemias. These chemicals can be potent even once-removed from those who work with them; the children of petrochemical workers have twice the incidence of developing leukemias. Even auto mechanics show higher than average incidence of bladder and kidney cancers.[3]

THE ASBESTOS CONNECTION

The name asbestos comes from the Greek word *asbesta* which means that it cannot catch fire. Asbestos is the generic name given to a series of minerals which are silky and fibrous in form. The fibers are tiny and almost invisible; two million of them can fit on the head of a pin.

The ancient Greeks knew of asbestos' fire resistant qualities and used it in lamp wicks and cremation cloths. Because of its strength and resiliency, they used it in the manufacture of pottery and textiles. But they also understood its potential dangers. Pliny the Younger, whose letters painted a vivid description of life and conventions in the Roman Empire, noted that people who worked with asbestos often became ill.

Because of these qualities—including strength, light weight, resistance to heat and fire, and ability to withstand chemical corrosion—asbestos was considered a "magic mineral," and its use in the 20th century spread like wildfire. In 1932, when the state-of-the-art cruise ship, the Queen Mary, was under construction, mock cabins were built and ignited to test different materials. Cabins utilizing asbestos-based boards established their supremacy in fire resistance. It is still used liberally in the manufacture of more than 3,000 commercial consumer products ranging from ships to portable hair dryers. The serious danger involved in its use is that asbestos, when it ages, begins to crumble and expels a fine, lethal dust.

Today, millions of people are in jeopardy because of exposure to these destructive dust particles, which can cause scarring in the lungs

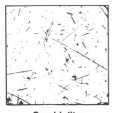
Crocidolite

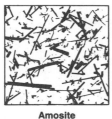
Amosite

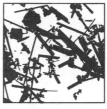
Anthophyllite

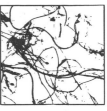
Chrysotile

Unlike chrysotile (white) fibers, which are curly and fine, those of the amphibole family (Crocidolite/blue), Amosite/brown, Anthophyllite), are straight and harsh. Crocidolite is considered the most deadly when inhaled.

Long, thin and not very soluble, crocidolite fibers are likely to reach the peripheral airways and remain ensconced. (Reprinted with permission from The Journal of Respiratory Disease, p.33, May 1986)

when inhaled, as well as cancers in many organs. The magic mineral of yesterday, this wonderful construction material of the 20th century, is becoming a nightmare for the present and future. In addition to its cost in human health, the surveillance of asbestos in the buildings and the schools will cost an estimated 100-150 billion dollars in the next decade for abatement and removal.[4]

Approximately one American dies every 59 minutes of asbestos-related problems, and 200,000 Americans will die from asbestos-related causes before the year 2000.[5] According to EPA estimates, between 3,300 and 12,000 new cases of cancer related to asbestos exposure are reported each year in the United States.[6]

Sources and Types

Raw asbestos is found in various soft rocks from which it is mined and milled throughout the world. Canada is the principal producer of asbestos in the western world, and other major producers are South Africa, the Soviet Union and China. About 90 percent in current use is white asbestos, the remaining ten percent is blue or brown. The blue variety, containing a high concentration of iron in its chemical structure, is far more lethal and was, unfortunately, used in ship construction during the Second World War.

DID YOU KNOW THAT?

- 850,000 metric tons of asbestos were used in 1973 in the United States, most in the form of sprayed building insulation.
- In that year, 50 asbestos manufacturers were listed in *Fortune 500*'s list of most prosperous United States companies.
- In 1985, 155,000 tons of asbestos were used in the United States. This marked decline in use is attributed to new EPA regulations. The province of Quebec, Canada, alone stands to lose 56 million dollars in revenue and up to 3,500 jobs in its asbestos mining industry.[7]

How Do We Get Exposed to Asbestos?

Dr. Irving Selikoff of the Mt. Sinai Hospital School of Medicine in New York has been a pioneer in the study of asbestos-related disease. His efforts have earned him the nickname "Dr. Asbestos." Dr. Selikoff has described the exposure to asbestos as occurring in three waves.

As mentioned before, raw asbestos is mined, milled and used in fabrication of different products such as cement, shingles, insulation, fabrics, and automobile brake linings. Those in the textile industries have had the highest degree of exposure, marking the first wave of exposure to asbestos.

Forming the second wave are those who work with and install asbestos products. The biggest occupational hazard comes from dust particles that are emitted during cutting, shaping and installing asbestos. Workers who use manufactured asbestos products, in building homes or offices, in automobile manufacture or in ship building, are at greater risk than the rest of the population. Included here are the countless numbers of "do-it-yourselfers" who get short but intense periodic exposures.

The popularity of asbestos as a construction material reached a peak during World War II and the subsequent post-war building boom. An alarming number of asbestos related diseases also peaked in the late 1950s and early 1960s. This prompted numerous studies in many countries where workers used asbestos products. In 1964, Dr. Selikoff did a landmark study on insulation workers in the New York and New Jersey metro areas where he established that asbestos is responsible not only for causing asbestosis, a disease which causes scarring in the lungs, but for many types of cancers, especially of the lung.[8] Later, similar studies were done on shipyard workers on the Virginia coast who were engaged in refurbishing old war ships. Much of their work involved ripping out old asbestos panels. These shipyard workers have shown an increased risk of lung cancer and many other cancers.

The third wave of exposure is the population in general—all of us. Aging asbestos crumbles into fine dust, and gets into air, water and food. When the asbestos fiber is airborne it knows no boundaries. Whether you work as a secretary in an asbestos factory, or you are the spouse of a factory worker who brings home heavy concentrations of asbestos in his/her clothing, you can be exposed to these particles of dangerous dust. If you live within a half mile of an asbestos factory, or any urban city, you have been exposed to a significant amount of asbestos fiber. Even a cow grazing near an asbestos factory was found to have asbestos in its lungs due to asbestos fiber air pollution in the area.

Asbestos has been used in the construction of thousands of public buildings—private homes, schools, hospitals, etc. According to EPA estimates there are 700,000 federal and commercial office buildings and apartment houses that contain asbestos. There are 100,000 to 200,000 private homes that contain asbestos in the easily crumbled form, mostly in the forced air and heating-and-cooling systems. It is flaking off and exposing millions of residents and workers.

Between 1950 and 1970 asbestos was commonly used as a fire proofing material in school construction. Nationwide, 31,000 schools have been found to have asbestos in the ceiling panels. Fifteen million children and 1.4 million school employees, especially janitors, are exposed to asbestos in these schools. It is estimated that 1.5 to three billion dollars will be required to remove this asbestos.[9]

Millions of seamen around the world are exposed to dangerously high levels of asbestos, as this material was a standard for ship construction for many years, used everywhere from boiler room insulation to toasters in the galley. The junk yards and millions of automobiles on the road have asbestos in clutch plates and brake linings. Service station attendants normally use compressed air to clean out the asbestos residue from brake drums, thus exposing themselves to dangerously high levels of the fiber.

Thousands of portable hair dryers as well as salon type hair dryers used asbestos for insulation, thus, 41,000 beauticians and barbers in the United States may be in the same high risk environment from using these appliances every day as shipyard workers and seamen. Even the sand in children's sandboxes has been found to be contaminated with asbestos.

Removing asbestos from or demolition of old asbestos contaminated buildings leads to very intense exposures, not only to the demolition workers but to the surrounding neighborhood as well. These days many contractors claim they are asbestos contractors, with a bucket and scraper in hand ready to collect this "white-gold." A contractor can make 100,000 dollars for cleaning up a medium sized school. Fortunately, there is a proper procedure for removing asbestos from a building set by EPA guidelines, so only certified contractors should be allowed.

These examples above illustrate the situations where asbestos can be inhaled into the lungs. However, this insidious material can be swallowed and get into the digestive tract. Asbestos contaminates water via many sources. In some areas, natural underground deposits contaminate the ground water. In other areas, lakes and rivers have been polluted by industrial dumping of asbestos waste.

Contamination can also occur when water is transported through cement pipes. Asbestos fibers also get into beer, wine and soft drinks; the filters used to strain these products contain asbestos. American beer has one to two million fibers per liter, Canadian beer four to six million fibers per liter, Italian vermouth has 11.7 million fibers per liter, and ginger ale has the highest asbestos fiber count with 12.2 million per liter. The drinking water near the Thetford Asbestos Mines in Quebec, Canada showed the incredible amount of 172.7 million fibers per liter because of natural contamination from underground deposits.[10]

The Consequences of Exposure to Asbestos

There is no "safe" level of exposure to asbestos, but the more intense and prolonged the exposure, the shorter it will take to develop an asbestos-related disease. People who have been exposed to asbestos by inhalation, develop scarring in the lungs, called asbestosis, ten to 20 years after exposure. Anyone exposed to asbestos can develop scarring in the lungs. This was recently confirmed by Drs. Irving Selikoff and Stephen Levin in a study coordinated by the New York School Board of Education on 660 school custodians. They found that 33 percent of the custodians had scarring in their lungs and this percent rose to 40 percent if the custodian had worked in schools for longer than 35 years. Paul Brodeur of the *New York Times* feels that what happened to construction workers who installed asbestos in schools (75 percent of them are dying of asbestos-related cancers) and the families of these workmen (30 percent of the wives and children exposed to the dust in their work clothes are suffering from asbestos-related illnesses) is also happening to school custodians and their families.

Initial studies on asbestos have shown that it causes high rates of lung cancer and mesothelioma, a cancer of the lining of the chest wall and abdominal cavity. Asbestos workers are normally at a ten times greater risk than the general population of developing lung cancer, and if they are smokers too, this risk multiplies to 90 times! Apparently the cancer-causing chemicals in tobacco smoke can gain entry into the cells more easily, assisted by the asbestos fibers.

There is suggestive evidence of asbestos causing many other cancers, including cancers of the larynx, esophagus, stomach, kidney, colon, and ovaries, and most recently eye cancers.[11] Asbestos has also been suspected as a cause of gastrointestinal cancer since asbestos-lined pipes are used for transporting water. Recently, a lymphatic cancer has been found in asbestos workers called "asbestos workers' lymphoma," and documented in an ongoing Cancer Surveillance Program in Los Angeles County.[12]

How to Protect Yourself

Since the mid 1970s much has been done to educate the public on the dangers of asbestos by both the EPA and the National Institute of Occupational Safety and Health (NIOSH). The process of phasing out asbestos use in commercial and consumer products and construction got under way in 1973 when, through the efforts of the EPA, asbestos insulation was banned from all new construction.

In 1986, the EPA proposed a ban on the use of the five most commonly used asbestos products such as: roofing, flooring felts, floor tiles, asbestos-cement pipes, and asbestos clothing. Efforts are underway to phase out asbestos completely.

Asbestos in Your Home

To confirm the presence of asbestos in your home, you can collect a sample of the suspicious pulverized material in a small container with an air-tight lid and send it to a specialized lab for analysis.

If you know for certain that there are asbestos ceiling panels in your home, they can be removed by a certified asbestos contractor. If removing them is too expensive, there are two other techniques. One method is to interfere with the flaking of the fiber by a process called encapsulation, which can be done by putting a paint-like sealer on the asbestos panels. Another method is by installing a dropped or false ceiling over the panels so that the crumbling fibers will not fall into the room.

Further information on asbestos can be received by calling the following agencies:

The Asbestos Whistle Blower's Hotline, 1-800-424-4000
The Asbestos Information System, (EPA), 1-202-475-7034
or call 1-800-334-8571 for a contact within your own state.

You can also refer to 1-800-424-9065 for EPA publications.

FIBERGLASS

Fiberglass is a synthetic fiber that is used in what is supposed to be a safer substitute for the natural fiber of asbestos. It is widely used as building material and as insulation in automobiles, furniture and packing, and in other appliances. Fiberglass is about a three billion dollar a year industry in the United States.

In general, exposure to any of the different types of fibers like asbestos, fiberglass, ceramics, and rock wool are hazardous. Synthetic fibers have been studied and the results appear to be similar to those of asbestos. These fibers get into the lungs and stay there. Studies on laboratory rats have shown increased rates of leukemia from exposure to synthetic fibers, and it is suspected that these fibers may also adversely affect the immune system. One study of 45,000 synthetic fibers workers in the United States and Europe has shown an increased rate of lung cancer as compared to the general population.

Synthetic fibers should be treated just like asbestos and all efforts should be made to minimize exposure to them.

SOOT, TARS AND OILS

As early as 1775, Percival Pott, an English physician, described a cancer of the skin of the scrotum which was prevalent among young chimney sweepers. He named it "chimney sweepers' cancer." Later on, it was discovered that the cancer-causing property of soot was due to a polycyclic hydrocarbon called Benzopyrene, a chemical found in soot and tar. Present-day steel and foundry workers are exposed to this chemical and show an increased incidence of this cancer and others of the lung and stomach.

We are all quite familiar with tar on our rooftops and roads and driveways. Tar is most commonly derived from distillation of coal as it is converted into coke. Many coal by-products-such as oils, paraffins, waxes, benzenes and creosotes—are obtained during the distillation process. Coal tar and its by-products were the mainstays of the chemical industry until petrochemicals took over in the 20th century. Even though coal tar as a basis for chemical industries has declined, coal tar based products are still widely available for consumer use: dandruff shampoos, tar ointment with sunlamp treatments for psoriasis (a skin condition), and other skin ointments. Patients who are on prolonged treatment for psoriasis with these medications have a higher incidence of skin cancer.

Creosote, a wood preservative, is used to treat wood for outdoor construction use. Treated wood should never be burned in indoor fireplaces as the chemical gives off carcinogenic fumes.

Coal tar pitch and asphalt are other by-products that are frequently used in roofing and road re-surfacing. There are an estimated 150,000 workers who use these products and they show higher than average incidence of lung and skin cancers.

Oils from coal tar products have carcinogenic agents similar to those of coal tar. Although to a lesser extent than in the past, workers in the textile and the tool and dye industries are still exposed to oil "mists," which are generated during hot metal cutting operations. These workers show higher than average incidence of skin, sinus and lung cancers. Preventive steps in this area include cleanliness and good hygiene as well as protective clothing for the workers.

PESTICIDES: A DANGEROUS DEPENDENCE

Pesticide is the generic name for the chemicals that are made toxic enough to kill different types of annoying pests that encroach on our lives. There are approximately 35,000 different formulations of pesticides that have been introduced since 1945, made from about 15,000 different compounds.[13] In the United States in 1985, farmers, home gardeners, contractors, pest control fumigators and exterminators, as well as the government, purchased four billion dollars worth of these products. Each is compounded to act generally upon specific pests: insecticides act upon insects; miticides act upon mites; herbicides act upon weeds and unwanted vegetation; and rodenticides act upon rodents and vermin.

It would be hard to imagine our present standard of life, social benefits, health and sanitation, and level of food supply without pesticides. Many of today's consumers, however, are not aware that there is a heavy cost associated with their use.

In 1984, the National Academy of Science released some disturbing findings: only ten percent of all pesticides available to United States consumers had been tested adequately for health assessment![14] Furthermore, 38 percent of these products contained no information on toxicity at all. According to the NIOSH report of October 1978, 27 of the pesticides should be controlled as suspected occupational carcinogens.

Unfortunately, the effects of pesticides do not stop with pests: they kill all forms of life, and should more properly be called "biocides." They can act acutely and cause accidental poisonings. Dr. Michael Loevinsohn at the Centre for Environmental Technology in London, writes that there have been occurrences of this throughout the world, killing more than 10,000 people annually.[15] Another hazard is the persistence of these chemical agents in the soil, causing water pollution and leaving pesticide residues on food long after it has been picked and shipped. The most important long-term hazard of these poisonous chemicals is their proven carcinogenic effects on laboratory animals and in human beings, even at low levels of exposure.

There have been three stages, or generations, of pesticides through history. The first generation, those that were in use up to World War II, were mostly salts of arsenic, lead, copper, zinc, and mercury. Extremely toxic compounds, these products presented great risks of pollution to the environment and increased risk of cancer to their users.

The second generation pesticides were a result of the development of the petrochemical industry during World War II. The first example in this category was the development of chlorinated pesticides like DDT. Later many other related chemical agents were developed for use as insecticides and weed-killers.

The third generation represents the intelligent use of these agents with botanical pesticides along with organic gardening called Integrated Pest Management.

DID YOU KNOW THAT?

- Over four billion kilograms of pesticides were produced in United States in 1984.[16]
- Out of these, 1.6 billion kilograms were herbicides, 1.5 billion insecticides, and the remaining were fungicides.
- Consumption has been increasing at the rate of five percent per year since 1982.
- 90 percent of these pesticides are synthetic compounds.

Insecticides

Botanical insecticides are used for small jobs around the garden or farm. Three chemicals, all extracts from plants, are most commonly used as the basis of these insecticides: nicotine, pyrethrum, and rotenone.

Inorganic insecticides, the most widely used of general insecticides, are made from the salts of heavy metals and non-metals. Arsenic is the most frequently used, especially in vineyards, and is associated with the risk of pollution and cancer.

Synthetic insecticides are made of compounds in three categories: chlorinated compounds, organophosphorus compounds, and carbamate compounds. Although not considered carcinogenic, organophosphate pesticides when used in combination with other pesticides can have a toxicity up to 50 times higher than when used alone. Chlorinated insecticides are the most important, especially because of their widespread use and the number of serious problems they create, as described in the following section.

The Wonder Chemicals — Chlorinated Compounds

DDT was hailed as a wonder chemical when it first appeared for commercial use in 1940 because a very small amount would go a long way in killing many kinds of insects. Its discovery as an insecticide was of such enormous importance throughout the world that Paul Mueller, the researcher, won a Nobel Prize in 1948. Besides increasing the productivity and yield of farms throughout the world by destroying pests, it eliminated the malaria-carrying mosquito in the tropics and did the same for other insects that carried diseases such as yellow fever and plague.

Rachel Carson's Warning

Another picture of DDT and its related compounds began to emerge about 1962. Rachel Carson's best-selling book *Silent Spring* painted a portrait of toxically overdosed fish, birds, and many friendly insects whose ecological chain had been short circuited. Widespread pollution of soil, streams and drinking water were the results of our indiscriminate use of insecticides such as DDT. Their persistent effects on the environment remain long after their original function is completed.

Acute accidental poisoning is one of the problems with DDT. One million watermelons had to be destroyed in California in 1985 when it was discovered that they had been sprayed with Aldicarb, an insecticide normally used only on cotton, beans and potatoes. Before the source of the poisoning was discovered, however, 1,400 people had become violently ill from eating the tainted watermelons. A bigger problem than acute poisoning is the chronic exposure to these chemicals—of manufacturers, users, and the unsuspecting public.

At first, these chemicals were considered magical and economical. Small amounts could effectively kill off a major infestation. But over the years, a "pesticide treadmill" developed; more and more pesticide was required to achieve the same effect as subsequent generations of insects become more resistant to the toxic chemicals.

Why are these chemicals resistant to the day-to-day methods of garbage disposal and erosion that dissolve so much else in nature? Because of their intense toxicity, anything they come into contact with in the environment is rendered sterile. After interaction with pesticides, there is little left in the soil or water to break these chemicals down and they linger on for many years.

These chemicals can also build up in the food chain to the point of concentration one million times greater than found in the environment naturally.[17] When smaller bugs are eaten by larger ones, and smaller fish are eaten by larger fish, the concentrations of insecticide chemicals within each organism doubles or triples hundreds and thousands of times in a process called biomagnification. Thus, the persistence of these chemicals in the air, water, and soil, leads to large residues of carcinogens in the food we eat, which eventually accumulates in the fatty tissues of the human body.

Cancer on the Farm

Pesticides are generally used by farmers in a combination of insecticides and herbicides. The use of pesticides on the farm is, in general, not carried out according to proper safety procedures; consequently, farm laborers and their families are exposed to the highly toxic chemicals. These cause not only cancers, but other problems such as sterility, birth defects and affected immune system in both animals and humans.

Twenty-seven pesticides are suspected or known carcinogens according to the EPA. DDT has been proven to be carcinogenic in laboratory animals, which led to a severe restriction on its use in the United States in 1972. For the same reason, Aldrin and Dialdrin were also removed from the market in the same year. Chlordane and Heptachlor were found to cause childhood brain tumors and leukemia in humans, and that has led to severe restriction of the use of these chemicals in termite control. Toxaphene, another generally used pesticide, was found to be carcinogenic in lab animals.[18]

In humans, many studies have shown increased cancer risk in the manufacturers and users of these pesticides, as well as in the general public. Farming communities in the United States and in other countries which use pesticides have a very high risk of many cancers. A study done by Dr. Dennis D. Weisenburger at the University of Nebraska Medical Center followed the agricultural use of chlorinated insecticides from 1950 to 1980, showing that lymphomas and leukemias in the area increased two to four times over that period.

Those engaged in the manufacture of pesticides are at high risk for many cancers. In 1976 the results of a study of 2,100 workers employed in chlorinated pesticide plants showed higher incidence of esophageal, stomach and lymphatic cancers. Employees of pest control companies in the United States were found to be at higher risk for lung cancer, according to a study done in 1976 by prominent researchers H.H. Wang and Brian McMahon.[19]

Users of these pesticides have similar problems. Studies of 3,800 licensed pesticide exterminators have shown up to three times higher risk for leukemia, brain tumors and lung cancers than the average population. Those at greatest risk, however, are not those who manufacture or use these pesticides, but the general public who are exposed through the food chain in both home and garden use.

The natural chain of events makes us *all* at risk of exposure to high levels of toxic insecticides. In the book *Circle of Poison*, David Wier and Mark Schapiro describe how chemicals such as Dialdrin, Chlordane, and Heptachlor, which are banned from use in the United States, are nonetheless, manufactured in this country. They are exported to many countries in South America, and then return to haunt us in foods that are shipped here from those countries for consumption. According to the book's statistics, one-half of the green coffee beans imported in the United States, and 13 percent of the beans and peppers imported from Mexico were found to be in violation of FDA pesticide standards upon arrival.[20]

Studies done in New Zealand, Hawaii, and Florida have shown that many lung cancer patients have shown higher than average levels of pesticide Dialdrin concentrations in their blood. Similar results have been seen in patients with leukemia and Hodgkin's disease as well.[21]

How to Minimize Your Exposure to Insecticides

The first step is to avoid using insecticides if at all possible. For home gardeners, crop rotation and crop alternation are some techniques that keep bug control at manageable levels. If you have to use an insecticide, you should make an intelligent use of these agents, A multi-step approach is called "integrated pest management." Organic gardening is one aspect of this current thinking on pesticide use.

Rotenone, nicotine and pyrethrum have been hailed as the "pesticides of the 1990s." They are all natural plant products and do not have the long term toxicity hazards of synthetic chemicals.

If an insecticide is necessary, either for termite treatment or for farming and gardening, it is best to avoid the "shot gun approach." Instead, identify the particular pest and use a narrow spectrum agent that is intended for its particular eradication. In farming and home gardening, the current emphasis is on keeping bugs and pests at a manageable level rather than wiping out the entire population. Beneficial insects like lady-bird beetles and lace-wing insects are now being used as natural predators to wipe out other pests.

Certified exterminators should always be called upon to apply insecticides. When an area has been sprayed, a warning sign should be posted for 72 hours, and pets and children not allowed near the area. It

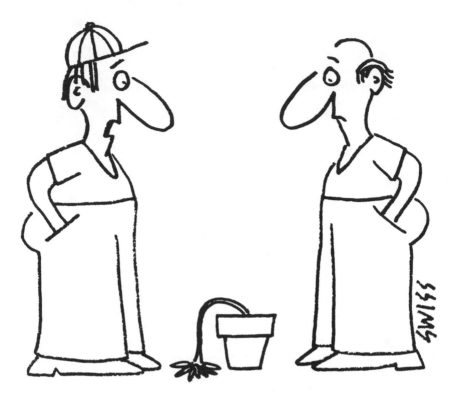

"I SPRAYED FOR APHIDS, CATERPILLARS,
BEETLES, FUNGUS AND MOLDS.
THE DACHSHUND NEXT DOOR GOT IT."
(Reprinted with permission from Thomas F. Wuthrich)

is better to avoid pesticide spraying professionals who guarantee that they will make your house "pest-free." They will have to use excess pesticide and in doing so will poison more than just the insects.

Last but not least, all insecticide containers should be treated as toxic waste, and therefore should not be put into the regular garbage. The ultimate goal is to have produce which is completely pesticide-free.

Further information about Integrated Pest Management can be obtained from:

Bio Integral Resource Center
P.O. Box 7414
Berkeley, California 94747.

Herbicides: The Greening of Suburbia and the Poisoning of America

Herbicides, or weed-killers, are agents that are directed at eliminating unwanted vegetation rather than unwanted pests and insects. Weed killers are used by everyone, from the government, the lawn care industry and farmers, to home gardeners.

There are a number of agents used as herbicides. Arsenic was one of the first, but its use has declined because of its extremely poisonous nature. It has been replaced by synthetic chemicals such as those of the chlorophenoxy group, the most famous of which is Agent Orange, used in Vietnam as a jungle defoliant. Others are in the Paraquat family, including dinitrophenols which is used frequently in spraying marijuana plants.

Agent Orange, a 50-50 mixture of 2,4-D and 3,4,5-T—all very toxic chlorinated compounds similar to DDT—caused a political stir and received much attention from the media when it was used in Vietnam. These agents are still being used in herbicide spraying in Oregon, and the controversy continues.

Home and garden use of herbicides is especially flagrant. There are 51 million home owners in the United States who take care of their own lawns, and the lure of a lush English garden and a healthy green lawn leads many of them to overdose in the use of weed killer. According to a 1980 study by the National Academy of Sciences, upscale suburban gardens and lawns in the United States are heavily saturated with herbicides as compared to farms. In 1984, private homeowners in the United States used 65 million pounds of herbicides on their lawns, about one-third of the total of non-agricultural pesticides used that year, according to EPA estimates.

Lawn care spraying services have become a big business in many communities. According to estimates of the Professional Lawn Care Association of America, lawn care companies now service approximately nine million households, for gross sales of 1.5 billion dollars annually. But there is an unpleasant side to this business. The compounds used are very poisonous, and some also have poisonous impurities like dioxin. Birth defects, miscarriages, and cancers are associated with people who manufacture or use these products.

There are many examples of cancer being caused by exposure to these agents: lymphoma rates are two to three times higher among Vietnam veterans who were in contact with Agent Orange; studies of different farming communities in the United States and in other countries such as New Zealand and Italy have shown that farmers have a much higher rate of lymphatic and leukemias, stomach, prostate, and bone marrow cancers; farmers in Iowa, Wisconsin, California and Nebraska have been studied, showing that they have consistently higher rates of cancer compared to rates in the general population.[22]

Recently a study done on Kansas farmers by Dr. S. K. Hoar and associates at the National Cancer Institute, showed an increased risk of six times more lymphatic cancer in farmers who were exposed to herbicides for 20 days in a year as compared to farmers with no exposure. Those farmers who actually mixed and applied the herbicides on the crops were at eight times increased risk. The study also showed that preventive measures in reducing the exposure would decrease the risk by 40 percent.[23] Prompted by this study, Chemlawn, a company that uses many products containing 2,4-D banned its use starting in 1987. The following pesticides have been banned or severely restricted and should not be used: DDT, Aldrin/Dieldrin, chlordane/heptachlor, 2,4,5-T, ketone, lindane, DBCP, mirex, silvex and toxaphene.

Farm laborers and their children are not the only ones at higher risk; eventually, we all eat herbicide-tainted food, putting us all at a high risk for cancer.

Fumigants and Sterilizing Agents

Ethylenedibromide (EDB) is a highly toxic cancer-causing agent, and was popularly used as a pesticide for citrus fruits and as a fumigant in grain silos and flour mills. In 1984, it was found in a variety of cornbread, cookie, cake and biscuit mixes, and these products were removed from the grocery shelves in several states. An even bigger hazard of EDB comes from automobile emissions, where it is used as an anti-knock agent in gasoline.

EDB has caused mutations, birth defects and tumors in lab animals in exceptionally short periods of time. Dr. Samuel Epstein, in an appearance on the TV show "Nightline," said that EDB is one of the most noteworthy carcinogens ever known and that he believes it is directly responsible for 3,000 cancer deaths annually in the United States.

Ethylene Oxide

Ethylene Oxide (EO) has been used since 1920 as a fumigant and sterilizing gas in hospitals. Approximately 75,000 health care workers are exposed to this chemical in the United States. Lab experiments on fruit flies and mice show this to be a cancer-causing agent. EO is suspected to cause leukemia and stomach cancer in the people who manufacture the chemical and those who work with it.

Fungicides and Wood Preservatives

In 1983, a rural family in Wisconsin unsuspectingly burned wood treated with chromium copper arsenate (CCA-50) in their fireplace. The accumulation of the heavy metals in the dust and ash in the home over two winters poisoned the whole family with arsenic and highly increased their lifetime risks of developing cancer. Creosote and arsenic are older wood preserving agents, but new synthetic chemicals have come along such as PCP (pentachlorophenol), a close chemical cousin to the herbicides, and hexachlorobenzene. Both are known carcinogenic chemicals.

A message to take home: do not reuse treated wood for burning in woodstoves and fireplaces. If you must use these agents as preservatives for wood to prevent rotting caused by fungus, use them with great caution and very sparingly. (*See also*, Creosote, Page 78)

BENZENE

Presently two million workers are exposed to benzene regularly.[24] One of the 12 most commonly used chemicals in this country, benzene is an important ingredient in tire manufacture. It is also an excellent solvent, and is used as an adhesive glue for the shoe industry, printing and publishing. It is an important intermediate in making different kinds of polishes, cosmetics, and other consumer products such as paint strippers and dry cleaning fluids. Small amounts of it often remain as an impurity in auto fuel, and levels of benzene are increasing now that lead is being removed from fuel to make it super-unleaded.

Millions of consumers are exposed to benzene whenever they use these benzene-tainted consumer products, and some school students use and misuse it in common lab experiments.

Most communities in the United States are exposed to benzene through automobile exhausts and gasoline fumes at gas stations. Chemical plants which manufacture benzene and coke oven plants also release significant quantities of benzene into the air. It has also been detected in cigarette smoke, in drinking water, and even in food stuffs.

About fifty years ago, a connection was made between benzene and the incidence of leukemia. Today it is well-known that workers who are exposed to benzene for four years have two times the risk of developing leukemia; those exposed five to nine years have 14 times the risk; and those exposed ten years or more have 33 times the risk. In experimental animals, benzene has been demonstrated over and over again to cause leukemia.

Many other kinds of cancer have been noted in humans from benzene, such as lymphomas and brain tumors in benzene workers. An alarming aspect of the increase in unleaded gasoline use is that although the amount of air pollution from lead drops, benzene increases and with it the leukemia rates. For the past ten years, rates of leukemia have gone up in service station workers and auto mechanics-according to a study of 40,000 death certificates in New Hampshire's Bureau of Disease Prevention.[25]

How to Protect Yourself from Benzene

Read labels. Products containing benzene should not be used or used minimally. There are alternative solvents available, such as Toluene and Xylene, but these also should be used sparingly as they contain benzene as a contaminant.

Pumping Gasoline

Gas station attendants are at a very high risk for exposure to petroleum and subsequently at increased risk for cancer. Benzene is three times heavier than air, so it sits on the top of the gas level in the tank. When you start pumping gas, benzene will be forced out of the fill opening. To prevent unnecessary exposure to benzene, avoid putting your head too close to the nozzle or the tank opening on your car. Also, avoid over-filling your tank. If your tank is slightly less than full, the benzene will not be forced out. Do not remove the nozzle from the gas tank until the remaining gas from it has been fully emptied. When you have finished filling the tank, close the tank opening immediately. Avoid gasoline spills on the ground, but if they do occur, they should be cleaned up with an absorbent material.

> *A Word of Caution to Gas Station Attendants:* Avoid skin contact with benzene-containing products. Benzene can be absorbed through the skin. Wear gloves and aprons. Workers have been known to clean their hands with gasoline and benzene, a very dangerous practice.

The State of California and many other states, including Michigan, now require a vapor recovery system on all of their gas pumps. It sucks the benzene out of the tank before it releases the fuel. It would be a good law for other states to adopt.

Truck drivers were also found to be at higher risk for cancer from their exposure to benzene. A study by Elaine Smith and colleagues at the University of Iowa shows that auto and truck mechanics also are at increased risk for bladder cancer.[26] Similarly, railroad workers are at increased risk from exposure to exhaust fumes.

The United States Occupational Safety and Health Administration has reduced acceptable workplace exposure levels from ten PPM (parts per million) to one PPM. It is estimated that a worker exposed to benzene at ten PPM for 40 years has an increased risk of leukemia of 154.5 times; this risk could be reduced to 1.7 times if the acceptable benzene exposure were reduced to one PPM.[27]

SOLVENTS

We have discussed one category of agents, benzene. Another category is chlorinated solvents, one of many types of solvents used in consumer products and industry. Chlorinated solvents are widely used in paints, industrial de-greasing and cleaning, automotive polishing and other products, adhesives, glues, dyes, polymers, plastics, textiles, printing inks, agricultural products and pharmaceuticals. Many people use chlorinated solvents at home in cleaning, arts, crafts, and hobbies. Because of their diverse uses, a large segment of the population is constantly exposed to them. According to a 1984 NIOSH report, 49 million pounds of industrial solvents were manufactured in the United States and 9.8 million workers were exposed to them through skin contact and inhalation.[28]

There are a number of agents used as chlorinated solvents. One such agent is trichloroethylene, widely used in de-greasing, aerosol propellants, and in solvents for dry cleaning. It has been shown to cause liver tumors in mice.[29]

In the past chloroform has been used as an anesthetic in hospital operating rooms, but is now used as a solvent. Recent research has shown that chloroform forms in hot showers and baths when the chlorinated water reacts with other organic impurities. To reduce the risk of exposure to chloroform, open a bathroom window or turn on an exhaust fan when bathing.

Methylene chloride is an aerosol propellant. It is used in paint strippers, hair sprays, de-greasing agents, pharmaceuticals and foods, and also in processing decaffeinated coffee and extracting fat. It is extremely toxic and has recently been proven to be carcinogenic in the liver and lungs of laboratory mice. An estimated one million people are exposed to methylene chloride in their workplaces.

Perchloroethylene is widely used in dry cleaning, fabric conditioning, and metal de-greasing. It is also used in home "do-it-yourself" dry cleaning preparations. There are 20,000 dry cleaning establishments and other industries that manufacture or use Perchloroethylene and it is currently being checked for its carcinogenic potential.

Carbon tetrachloride is used in the manufacture of freon for refrigerators and as a de-greasing agent. Rubber, leather and chemical industries, as well as pharmaceutical companies, also use carbon tetrachloride.

Ten billion pounds of Ethylene dichloride were used in 1973. It is among the highest volume chemical to be used in the United States, often to remove lead from gasoline. It is also suspected to be a carcinogen.

"Dry cleaned" clothes directly from the cleaners should be aired out at home in the garage or outside as they carry some residue solvent in them. A tip for "do-it-yourselfers": make your own spot removers. An all purpose spot remover can be made from ¼ cup borax plus two cups cold water, or from glycerine in undiluted vinegar. For fruit and tea stains, wash with boiling water.

FORMALDEHYDE: INDICTED AS CAUSE OF CANCER

Formaldehyde is a chemical with diverse uses. It is found in products such as nail polish, antiperspirants, permanent press clothes, mattresses, carpeting and tobacco smoke. In a foam state, it is used in homes as spray-on insulation, and is commonly used as a preservative for body parts or specimens in morgues and labs. An estimated eight billion pounds is used in the United States annually, either as a foam, as an adhesive mixed with urea and water to form a resin, or as a liquid called formalin.[30]

Formaldehyde as Insulation and Adhesive

Widely used as a home insulation material in the 1940s and early 1950s, formaldehyde was banned by the EPA in 1982, when it was found that it emitted dangerous fumes.

Another popular use of formaldehyde is as an adhesive in plywood and pressed wood products like particle board, frequently used in construction of mobile homes. Mobile homes are more prone to indoor air pollution because they tend to be more air tight than conventional houses. In the mid-1970s physicians coined the name "mobile home disease" to describe the diverse complaints that many mobile home dwellers were presenting, such as: sore throats, headaches, eye irritation. By 1977 researchers traced these complaints to formaldehyde fumes. Unfortunately, these fumes can come from insulation foam, especially when it is heated and the formaldehyde is liberated from the resin state (called "outgassing").

In a study done on 50 homeowners who filed their concerns with the Rocky Mountain Poison Center about formaldehyde as insulation, only 38 percent could *smell* the formaldehyde odors in their homes—consistent with the phenomenon of adaptation to odors. Presently, 11 million

90

mobile home dwellers in the United States are exposed to these noxious fumes every day, as are those people living in 500,000 conventionally built homes that use this material as insulation.[31]

Researchers are still unclear about the extent of cancer risk from formaldehyde exposure. Richard Hefter, an EPA official who headed a study of formaldehyde in 1987, estimates that two lifelong mobile home residents out of 10,000 will be afflicted with cancer caused by formaldehyde.[32]

Formalin, the liquid form of formaldehyde, is used as a disinfectant in hospital labs and as a preservative for tissue specimens and embalming. Dialysis patients use formaldehyde for disinfecting kidney machines, and college students are routinely exposed to the chemical in labs. Embalmers, who frequently use formaldehyde, are at an increased risk for skin, kidney and brain cancers according to a study published in the *International Journal of Cancer.*[33]

The highest levels of exposure to formaldehyde are in the garment industry where 777,000 workers were exposed to relatively high levels regularly.[34] Recent studies have shown that these workers have two to three times the risk of lung, nose and sinus cancers, as anticipated from earlier animal lab studies. A 1986 EPA study conducted in Seattle by Dr. Thomas Vaughan at the University of Washington showed that formaldehyde exposure was linked to a rare throat cancer called Nasopharyngeal cancer.

An occupational survey determined that 1.6 million Americans were in contact with formaldehyde in their place of work,[35] but its widespread use in consumer and household products puts us all at risk.

How to Prevent Exposure to Formaldehyde

If your home was insulated before 1970, chances are that formaldehyde foam was not used. Some local and state health departments will conduct tests at little or no charge to homeowners. If the formaldehyde level is determined to be "unsafe," there are some less expensive steps of prevention short of removal (which can run up to 20,000 dollars in most homes):

1) Seal all cracks in the walls;
2) Apply two coats of barrier vapor paint to the walls—it seals off half of the fumes and is good for a couple of years;
3) Apply mylar or vinyl wallpaper to the walls. Butyl or acrylic latex caulking, weatherstripping or special foam backed tapes can be used to seal the junctions of floor and walls where air can leak and send fumes into the home. The most effective barrier is aluminum foil. Formaldehyde fumes can't cross foil.[36]

When buying furniture and panelling at home, buy goods made with solid wood; even plywood is better than particle board because it does not "out-gas" as much formaldehyde. For home insulation buy fiberglass insulation instead of foam.

If none of the above methods are feasible, you can at least open windows. A good sized air filter can help to reduce formaldehyde fumes. Most interesting of all, a spider plant grown in the house can absorb most formaldehyde fumes. Two plants of chlorophytum elatum in one gallon containers will purify a house of about 1,800 square feet—but just one will also help.

Formaldehyde monitors are available so that you can check the level in your home. Below are the address of two companies that can be contacted for more information:

3M Center
OH and S Products Division
Building 227-7 West
St. Paul, Minnesota 55144
   (612) 733-1110

OR

E.I. Du Pont de Nemours and Company, Inc.
Applied Technology Division
Clayton Building, Concord Plaza
Wilmington, Delaware 19898
   (302) 764-2798

DYES

History of the Dye Industry

Physicians knew before the turn of the 20th century that workers exposed to dyes or dye intermediates were at risk for developing bladder cancer. The story of dyes took a sensational turn when a British angling champion died of bladder cancer at age 41, purportedly just from touching dyed earthworms.[37] The case indicated that the dyes got into the body through the skin.

The dye industry is a solid example of doing human experimentation in the causation of cancer. As early as 1895 a German surgeon named Rehn noted increased bladder cancer in dye workers, and it was thought that the dyes contained a carcinogenic agent. The German workers who produced magenta from aniline, a dye intermediate, were developing high rates of bladder cancer. The aniline was suspected of causing the bladder cancer, called "aniline cancers." Later research pointed to another dye intermediate called betanaphthylamine as the causative agent of bladder tumors in dye workers.

Long latency periods of disease from dyes are common—usually 18 years or more. It is estimated that 50 to 60 percent of human bladder cancers can be caused by industrial exposure to dyes.[38]

Types of Dyes

There are three basic categories of dyes: those used in food products, those used for human hair, and industrial dyes. This section deals only with industrial dyes. Food and hair dyes are explored in detail later in this chapter.

Dyes are used in a variety of different industries. Industrial dyes may be used in rubber, textile, printing, leather, paints, or paper. Benzidine based dyes have been proven to be a human and animal carcinogen, especially causing bladder cancer.[39] Two such benzidine dyes, direct blue six and direct black 38, have been known to cause hepatocellular cancer and liver tumors. In a study on Japanese kimono painters who came into contact with benzidine dyes, bladder cancers developed at higher than normal rates.[40] Benzidine based dyes are used quite extensively. According to NIOSH, 3.3 million pounds of the dyes are used in 63 occupations and 79,000 workers are exposed to them.

Related Occupations

Fishermen have also worked with dyes when they use stains for maggot bait. Dyes used most often among this group are auramine, rhodamine and chrysoidine, in red and yellow colors, all of which have been linked to cancers in animals. Some studies have suggested that cancers of the urinary tract in these fishermen could be related to exposure to these dyes. Two doctors at the Queen Elizabeth Hospital in Birmingham believe that approximately one million people in England alone have been exposed to dyed earthworms.[41] I strongly recommend that these dyed worms should not be handled without gloves and should not be touched at all by children. Many children take up the sport of fishing, and caution should be used to protect them from this potential exposure.

ARTIFICIAL RUBBER AND PLASTICS

Before World War II, rubber was made from rubber trees located in South America and the Philippines. As these supplies became unreliable during the war, demand at home increased. Necessity being the mother of invention, scientists found a way to synthesize this vital material. Unfortunately, because of the multiple exposures to workers, the risk of lung, stomach, bladder cancers and leukemias increased.

A chemical named Butadiene was used in the initial process. Later on the process became much more complex. A large number of other chemicals, including solvents such as benzene, hardening agents, stabilizers, asbestos, dyes and paints were added to the manufacture of artificial rubber to make other products. Vinyl chloride was one such chemical, and acrylonitrile was another. Styrene was incorporated for making styrofoam, and vinyl acetate was added to make textiles. These chemicals could be combined to make other products.

Plastics can be placed into two categories: thermolabile and thermostable. The thermolabile are soft plastics in which the monomers (a molecular unit of a polymer) do not have a strong bond and can leach into foods stored in soft plastics, especially in combination with heat such as in hot weather or in microwave use. Alternatively, thermostable plastics have a strong bond between monomers and can withstand heat well, so the danger of pollution is greatly reduced. Thus consumers must be concerned with these materials. Some of the original chemicals in these products can leach into food in containers made of them. An example is a case in the 1970s, where hundreds and thousands of plastic soft drink bottles had to be destroyed because the chemicals in the plastic were leaching into the beverage in high concentration.

Plastics are not biodegradable. They remain in the environment for a long time and should be recycled.

COMMON POLLUTANTS: DIOXINS, PBBs AND PCBs

A number of chemical pollutants like PCBs, PBBs and dioxins are present in the air, water, soil, and the food we eat, and eventually they will appear in our body fat, the final junkyard. Other pollutants are polycyclic hydrocarbons in smoke, tar, soot and petrochemicals. Asbestos and pesticides, also considered pollutants, were described earlier in this chapter. Waste oil is also an important source of pollution; it led to the unhappy demise of the town of Times Beach, Missouri, in 1983, as described below.

Dioxins and Dibenzofurans

Dioxins are one of the most toxic compounds known to mankind. They form as unintended contaminants in the production of different chlorinated hydrocarbons like 3,4,5-T, which is a weed killer, and TCP, which is trichlorophenol. These agents are used in forestry for weed control and as a defoliant. Lumberjacks and paper mill workers are exposed to these agents, especially in the production of wood pulp. A number of studies have been done on Vietnam veterans and Swedish forestry workers who were exposed to Agent Orange, a 50-50 mixture of 3,4,5-T and 2,4-D.

In 1983 there was a mixup in Times Beach, Missouri when used oil, containing dioxin, was mixed with sludge from another facility, producing hexachlorophene. It was sprayed over the dirt roads of Times Beach as a dust control measure. When the rains came, the dioxin present in the waste oil contaminated the whole town, and Times Beach had to be evacuated.

Dioxin has also been found in cigarette smoke and, in general, is contained in trace amounts in most fires. Very large amounts of dioxin and dibenzofurans are produced when PCBs burn. In a 1981 fire of the Binghamton Tower office building in New York State, the entire 14 floors of the building were completely polluted. They were considered uninhabitable because the transformers containing oil and PCBs had burned during the fire.

Similarly, exposures to dioxin have occurred in the production and use of compounds such as 3,4,5-T and trichlorophenol. Occupational exposures have occurred through accidents at the work place. Studies have been done on 3,4,5-T production workers, and Swedish forestry workers showing a five times higher risk of soft tissue sarcomas.[42] Farmers who have used these products have shown an increased rate of cancers, especially lung cancer, ovarian cancer, soft tissue sarcomas, non-Hodgkin lymphoma, and Hodgkin's Disease. Dioxin has also been suspected to be extremely toxic to the immune system and a cause of miscarriages and birth defects.

Most of the notoriety for dioxin came from the Vietnam veterans, who got heavy exposure when Agent Orange was mixed with oil and sprayed from the air to uncover the jungle hideouts of the Viet Cong. Recent studies have shown that the Vietnam veterans have higher rates of cancer.

PBBs

PBB is used mainly as a fire retardant. Widely used in the early 1970s, an accidental contamination in Michigan brought the dangers of this chemical to the public's attention. In 1973, bags of the fire retardant became mixed up with cow feed at a factory. Thousands of cows, representing hundreds of thousands of pounds of meat and gallons of milk, had to be slaughtered—the most costly contamination ever to occur in the United States agriculture industry. Dr. Mary Wolff and her associates at the Environmental Sciences Laboratory of Mt. Sinai School of Medicine have demonstrated that PBB is carcinogenic in laboratory animals.[43]

PCBs

PCB, an oil-like chemical, has been used in various industries since 1930. Its major use has been in electrical transformers for transferring energy and capacitors for storing electrical charges. PCBs have also been used for sealants and insulators in televisions and as components of copying paper and fluorescent lights.

In 1979 the EPA banned the use of this chemical in the United States because it was found to cause liver cancer in laboratory animals.[44] In the meantime, PCB has polluted everything it contacts: air, water, soil, food, even human bodies. It is estimated by Dr. Richard Fruncillo of the Jefferson Medical College in Philadelphia that more than one million workers have been exposed to PCBs, especially those who worked in repairing broken technological equipment.[45] But the biggest danger is still to come: old transformers will be dumped or disposed of carelessly in junkyards across America, having the potential to affect entire populations adversely. They have already started leaking, beginning the ecological process of biomagnification through rain water. Traces of this chemical have already appeared in samples of human breast milk.

MISCELLANEOUS OCCUPATIONAL EXPOSURES

AGENTS	USES AND EXPOSURE	RELATED CANCERS
ARSENIC	Insecticides and Wood Preservatives. Medicinal use in the past. Pigment like Schele's Green. Cementing and refining of ore causes air pollution. Water pollution from natural deposits in the ground.	Skin Liver Lung
COBALT	Alloys for rustproofing, paints and pigments like cobalt blue.	Lung and Connective Tissue
NICKEL	Used in alloys for making stainless steel, electronics and coins, batteries. Plating and welding. Public exposure from auto exhaust and cigarette smoke.	Nose Sinus

AGENTS	USES AND EXPOSURE	RELATED CANCERS
CADMIUM	Used for alloys, electroplating welding, pigments, alkaline batteries and many other uses in metallurgy. Public exposure by inhalation of urban air from smelters and cigarette smoke.	Respiratory Prostate Testicular
LEAD	In storage batteries, paints and pigments. Pottery and ceramics. B.B. ammunition pellets. Pesticides, solders and casting. Air pollution from zinc and lead smelters pose a risk to the whole community. Water pollution from lead soldering in pipes. Bone meal has high lead concentration. Auto exhaust is an important source of lead air pollution.	Brain Kidney Leukemia
CHROMIUM	Used in chrome plating, alloys for steel, paints, and pigments and leather tanning.	Lung
BERYLLIUM	Used for alloys in nuclear industry, space vehicles, X-ray tubes and fluorescent lights.	Lung
IRON ORE	Hematite mining, iron ore mining, exposure high in foundry workers.	Lung
LEATHER	Multiple exposures in the tanning and dyeing processes.	Bladder Oral Pharynx Larynx
WOOD	Multiple exposures in the logging of wood-like weed killers and in sawing and pulp making and in carpentry work.	Lymphatic Soft Tissue
TEXTILES	The main exposure in the textile industry is the excessive use of formaldehyde and in the printing and dyeing of textiles.	Nasal Cavity and Lung

COSMETICS, HAIR DYES, AND TALCUM POWDER

Gray Areas for the Consumer

In the eyes of the United States government and its regulatory agencies, a cosmetic improves appearance whereas a drug diagnoses, relieves, or cures a disease. There are gray areas where these distinctions get blurred. Dandruff shampoos, antiperspirants, sun tanning preparations with sunscreen, lotions and emollients containing hormones, and anti-baldness preparations are just a few examples.

Possible Carcinogenic Ingredients in Cosmetics

Many cosmetic products commonly used by the average consumer contain ingredients that may be carcinogenic. Below is a list of some such ingredients.

Saccharin: a sweetener in toothpaste.

Toluene: a solvent in nail polishes and polish remover.

Artificial colors: Blue #1 used in facial creams, cosmetics, perfumes and lotions.

BHT: used in lipsticks, shaving cream, and other skin care products.

Coal Tar: used in dandruff shampoos.

DEA: used in hair conditioners and may form nitrosamines. It is made with ethylene oxide and both chemicals are suspected carcinogens.

Formaldehyde: used in eye make up, nail polish (up to five percent), shampoos, mouthwashes, deodorizers. Also a common ingredient of hair spray and styling mousse. Some dandruff shampoos may contain formaldehyde (an easy substitution is to rub baking soda into the hair).

Iron Oxide: a colorant in eye make-up.

Talc: Feminine deodorants have talc which is often contaminated with asbestos and has been linked with ovarian cancer.

The rules regulating drug manufacture and sales of cosmetics are very different. The FDA requires every drug manufacturer to register once a year and update its lists of current products twice yearly. With cosmetics, all such registration is voluntary. Contrary to most Americans' notions, no cosmetic needs a review from the FDA before it becomes available to the public. Anyone can go into the cosmetic business.

The American cosmetic industry grossed 15 billion dollars in 1980 and produced 25,000 products, containing a total of 8,000 ingredients.[46] Administrators with the FDA claim that they have data on ingredients for no more than 20 percent of the cosmetic products on the market at any given time, and only four percent of these have filed experience reports. Animal studies, which may cost as much as 300,000 dollars to test one ingredient thoroughly, are not undertaken eagerly by most companies. Furthermore, the FDA can take action only "after the fact"—when a product has been proven to be harmful or after a certain number of customer complaints.

The rationale that allows this situation to exist was an outmoded theory that the skin formed a nearly perfect barrier that prevented chemicals from penetrating to the body. However, currently transdermal delivery of medications, or placing the drug on an adhesive disc which is slowly absorbed into the system, has become increasingly popular for treatment of seasickness and angina and will probably be utilized in many more ways in the future.

What degree of absorption is there when a foundation is left on the face for 12 hours; or when a lotion is spread over the entire body for tanning; or a hair color is massaged into the scalp every six weeks over the course of a lifetime?

Hair Dyes

It has been estimated that more than 33 million Americans dye their hair. Three types of dyes exist: natural, metallic and synthetic. Natural dyes such as henna are unpredictable in their results. Metallic dyes such as lead chromate are toxic to the body. Both natural and metallic dyes have been replaced by synthetic ones. Synthetic hair dyes are suspected of causing cancer.

Beauticians apply a variety of products to the hair as it is dyed. These include the dye itself, the oxidizer, hair conditioners, color modifiers, antioxidants, stabilizers, and other compounds. Although it is difficult to establish a definite cause and effect relationship between hair dyes and cancer, hairdressers and barbers have been found to be at higher risk for many cancers, including those of the breast and bladder. These reports led to the FDA warning on some permanent hair dyes

99

about their possible effects on the human body: "Warning: contains an ingredient that can penetrate your skin and has been determined to cause cancer in animals." In addition, caution with these dyes has been recommended by the American Cancer Society.

DID YOU KNOW THAT?

- More than 33 million Americans use hair dyes to lighten, brighten and cover gray in their hair, a total of 280 million dollars in annual retail sales.
- Approximately ¾ of these permanent dyes contain 2,4-diamino-anisole, which is also used in dyeing furs? This product is not manufactured in the United States, but imports of 2,4-diaminoan-isole are on the order of 25,000 pounds per year.[47]
- Tests done by the National Cancer Institute indicate that this and five other hair coloring ingredients are carcinogenic in rats. About 400,000 workers in the United States have potential exposure to 2,4-diaminoanisole, with barbers and cosmetologists comprising the greatest number.
- Among hairdressers, elevated proportional morbidity ratios (based on United States Department of Social Security disability awards made to female workers between 1969 and 1972) were observed for cancer of the digestive organs, respiratory system, breast and genital organs.

An English study showed an excess of breast cancer among single women hairdressers in the occupational mortality analyses of the Registrar General between 1959-1963. A University of California study on 58,000 hairdressers, manicurists, and cosmetologists, aged 20 to 62, found that they developed multiple myeloma at four times the rate of the general population. Of course, hairdressers come into contact with many chemicals, and this study implicated everything from hair dyes to shampoos and polish remover.[48]

How to Minimize the Risks from Dyes

From data acquired by NIOSH (the National Institute of Occupational Safety and Health), it appears that 2,4-diaminoanisole (MMPD) penetrates the skin and thereby enters the system. Thus skin contact with the chemical should be avoided in the workplace. Hairdressers should always wear rubber gloves when working with these preparations. Women who are concerned about the risks of hair dyes can color their hair by frosting or streaking processes which do not touch the scalp. Blonding, a process which bleaches the hair and then adds blonde color with a toner, is another procedure that is safer, for most toners do not contain the five suspected dyes. Henna, a vegetable dye, has no cancer risk but is less predictable in its results.

Talcum Powder

Like hair dyes, talcum powder has been connected to higher-than-average cancer risks. Talcum powder, a widely used product among both sexes and all age groups, has been cited since 1960 as a possible carcinogen. The first instance was a connection between the use of talc by surgeons on their surgical gloves and an increase in granulomas of the internal organs.

Pure talcum powder is not thought to be a cause of cancer, but Dr. T.K. Ng of the University of Sydney found that in many instances it is contaminated with asbestos fibers, which would make it a possible carcinogen.[49] In a Boston study done by Dr. Daniel Cramer, talc was linked to ovarian cancer risk over three times greater among women using talcum powder routinely on their sanitary napkins and genitals than women who did not.[50]

Talc is a popularly used component ingredient in many eye shadows and blushes. The 1972 study done by the Office of Product Technology of the FDA showed that 39 out of 40 talcums tested contained one percent asbestos fibers. The manufacturers have since claimed to have corrected this problem, but asbestos and talc fibers are similar in composition. Cornstarch, ricestarch, flour or white clay can be used in its place.

HOUSEWORK — A CANCER HAZARD

Perhaps this is the news that many housewives have been waiting for. Housework, along with the unanimous agreement on its drudgery and tedium, also carries a certain amount of risk to your health. University of Oregon researchers discovered by chance that housewives are at twice as much risk of dying from cancer as compared to the general population. I believe it is just a matter of time before the surgeon general will give it the proper notice. The present day broom closet has much in common with a chemical lab.

We all want a good lifestyle, and we have all accepted the Madison Avenue value system of clean and orderly houses that appear effortless to achieve. In recent years, as more women work outside the home, there is less time and inclination to spend on daily housecleaning tasks. To meet these needs and expectations, there has been an explosion of consumer cleaning products saturated with chemicals to solve problems such as ring around the collar, toilet-bowl ring, watermarks on glasses, high-shine floors and the like.

Many of these chemicals have not been adequately tested for carcinogenicity, and we are using them as if they were going out of style, and often quite carelessly. Proper precaution should be taken in the use of many of these products, and for some, use should be minimized or substituted with safer ingredients. Among the worst examples are carpet cleaners, spot removers, dry cleaning fluids (especially for silk and wool), and do-it-yourself dry-cleaning preparations that usually contain chlorinated solvents and petroleum distillation products.

Practical Household Alternatives

The following are some alternatives for the more commonly used household cleaning products that contain carcinogenic chemicals:

KITCHEN AND BATHROOM CLEANING

Glass cleaner: Two tablespoons of vinegar to one quart of water.

Toilet bowls: Substitute ½ cup of bleach.

Drain cleaner: Boiling water, followed by a plunger and/or plumber's snake.

Air freshener: get rid of the unwanted odors by opening windows and turning on a fan. Also, empty the garbage daily. A *pot pourri* which has a natural scent such as ground cloves and peppermint will work to "freshen" the air. Setting out some vinegar in an open dish also works.
Synthetic air fresheners are actually air polluters containing formaldehyde and many other petrochemicals.

Oven cleaner: make a paste of salt, baking soda and water, and apply with elbow grease.

LIVING AND DINING ROOM CLEANING

For wool or synthetic plush *carpeting*: pour sparkling soda water directly on the soiled area and blot dry with a towel.

Furniture polishes contain benzene derivatives. In their place, substitute 1 teaspoon lemon oil in one pint of mineral oil or rub crushed raw nuts on the wood as an oily polish.

For *polishing silver*, soak silver pieces in a quart of warm water with one teaspoon baking soda and one teaspoon salt and a piece of aluminum foil.

PLANTS AND PET CARE

Fleas: bathe and comb your pet frequently. An easy way to kill fleas is to heat your home to 122° F for several hours. Feed pets with brewers yeast which gives odor to the skin that fleas don't like. Commercial pet flea collars contain carbaryl. Lice shampoos for pets contain lindane. Both are pesticides with carcinogenic risk. Other pet products used for pesticide control contain arsenic, malathion, and methoxychlor. Proper precaution should be taken in their use and preferably not used at all.

Roach sprays: a substitute is to use chopped bay leaves and cucumber skins and boric acid in the cracks in the room, or set out a dish with one part baking soda and one part brown sugar.

Instead of using an *insecticide* for house plants, spray soapy water on the leaves and wipe off.

Rat and mouse killers: use a cat or a mouse trap instead of pesticides. "Rodent proof" your home by blocking rodent entries into your home (consult a pest control company).

Ants: wipe the area with a wet cloth. Spray hot peppers where the ants appear to come from. To keep ants away, sprinkle red chili pepper around the foundation of the house. Bay leaves in cupboards will also deter ants.

Lice shampoo: normally lindane is used, but the problem can be taken care of easily by using coconut oil as a shampoo alone with soap and water and a comb to pick out lice.

Food storage pests: (beatles, weevils, moths, mites) Prevention is the key. Inspect groceries carefully at the store, because that is where the pests come from. Store foods in containers with tightly closed lids.

Mothballs: you can prevent moths by spreading newspapers around the closet, or you can store clothes in a cedar chest or cedar closet or place cedar chips around the clothes.

ARTISTS AND HOBBYISTS: PLAYING WITH CARCINOGENS

Many people are involved in a variety of arts, crafts and hobbies at home. Many of these activities, from painting to working with photographic processes, involve applications of a multitude of chemicals containing asbestos, cadmium, chromium, magenta, benzene, chlorinated solvents and formaldehyde. Because many of these hobbies take place throughout the house, the entire family is at risk for exposure. Unfortunately, people are not educated in the safety measures necessary to prevent such exposures.

Potentially carcinogenic chemicals can be inhaled, swallowed or absorbed through the skin. Researchers recommend that hobby enthusiasts should ventilate the work area and work near windows, especially when spraying, plate making, silk screen painting and washing. In addition, the body should be protected by proper work clothes offering adequate skin protection, protective creams, goggles and gloves.

After working with arts and crafts materials, wash the skin thoroughly and launder work clothes separately from regular clothing. Eating and drinking should not occur when working with arts and crafts. If exposure is excessive, the workers should use a fan system and adhere to strict housekeeping measures to ensure that the chemicals do not remain and further contaminate the house. The hobbyist should also take extra time to read warning labels and instructions on how to use these chemicals. Retired people often devote the extra time they have to arts and crafts, and they expose themselves to a variety of chemicals in the process. Retired persons may not have the ability of a young person to tolerate a high exposure to certain chemicals such as benzene and formaldehyde. Physicians recommend that they need to be more cautious and take all precautions possible.

The following are examples of activities which we do in the home.

Painting: Painters come across a number of toxic compounds, including pigments containing heavy metals like lead, arsenic, cadmium, chromium, and mercury. They are also exposed to solvents, some dyes and hardening agents.

Ceramics and Pottery: People who work with ceramics are exposed to both colors and glazes that can contain nickel, cadmium, chromium and even uranium.

Sculpture and Casting: People involved in sculpture and casting are exposed to asbestos, wood dust and even formaldehyde. Metal casting leads to exposure to metal fumes and formaldehyde.

Jewelry Making and Welding: Jewelers are exposed to cadmium fumes. Welding fumes also contain nickel and ultraviolet light exposure. If solvents are nearby, deadly phosphine gas can be produced.

Plastics: People who work with different kinds of plastics are exposed to potentially dangerous monomers when the plastic is heated. Some examples are polyvinyl chloride, acrylic, glues, polyurethanes, fiberglass, polyester or epoxy resins. Plastics should not be heated or burned.

Woodworking: is hazardous because of the dust, glues and adhesives involved, which contain many carcinogenic chemicals.

CHAPTER FIVE NOTES

1. Janet M. Scarlett-Kranz, et al. "Urinary Mutagens in Municipal Waste Workers and Water Treatment Workers," *American Journal of Epidemiology.* Vol. 124, #6, 1986

2. Samuel Epstein, and J. Swartz, "The Fallacies of Lifestyle Cancer Theories," *Nature Magazine.* Vol. 289 (January, 1981)

3. *National Institute of Safety and Health,* Publication #657-012/325, (1977)

4. Brooke Mossman, and J. Bernard Gee, *New England Journal of Medicine,* (June 1989)

5. Annette Allerhand, and Edwin Flatto, *The Unseen Peril in Our Environment — Asbestos,* Plymouth Press

6. L. Moerwald, "Pushing Asbestos," *Environmental Action,* Nov/Dec. 1986

7. *Ibid.*

8. Victor Archer, J.Dean Gilliam, Joseph Wagoner, "Respiratory Diseases Mortality Among Uranium Miners," *Annals of New York Academy of Medical Sciences*

9. *American Medical News,* Sept. 1984

10. Allerhand and Flatto, *Unseen Peril: Asbestos*

11. *New England Journal of Medicine,* June 1989

12. *Medical Tribune,* Nov. 1982

13. John Davies, "Changing Profile of Pesticide Poisoning," *New England Journal of Medicine,* (March 26, 1987)

14. Rachel Carson Council, *Pesticides in Contract Lawn Maintenance,* (1984)

15. Michael Loevinsohn, *Lancet,* (June 1987)

16. F. Ebert, *Occupational Medicine,* (Year Book Medical Publishers, 1988)

17. S. Epstein, *The Politics of Cancer,* (New York: Anchor Books 1979)

18. "Cancer Epidemiology of Pesticide Manufacturers, Formulators and Users," International Agency for Research on Cancer *Monograph,* Vol. 30

19. H.H. Wang, and Brian McMahon, *Occupational Medicine,* (1976)

20. David Wier, and Mark Schapiro, *Circle of Poison,* Institute for Food Development Policy.

21. Epstein, *Politics of Cancer*.

22. IARC *Monograph* Vol. 30

23. Hoar, S.K., et. al., "Agricultural Herbicide Use & Risk of Lymphoma and Soft Tissue Sarcoma," *Journal of the American Medical Association*, Vol. 256, #9 (Sept. 5, 1986)

24. *NIOSH*. 1977

25. *Health and Environmental Digest*, (Oct. 1987)

26. E. Smith, "Toxic Art," *American Journal of Public Health*, (1985)

27. *New England Journal of Medicine*, (April 1987)

28. "Organic Solvents in the Workplace," *Journal of the American Medical Association*, Vol. 257, #23 (June 1987)

29. *Casarette & Doull's Toxicology*, p. 84-138 (New York: Macmillan Publishing Company, 1980)

30. Robert E. Hyatt, "Formaldehyde Exposure - A Case in Point," *Mayo Clinic Proceedings*, Vol. 59 (1984)

31. *Ibid.*

32. Richard Hefter, *Detroit News*, (April 1, 1987)

33. *International Journal of Cancer*, Vol. 31, (1983)

34. Eliot Marshall, "EPA Indicts Formaldehyde, 7 Years Later," *Science*, Vol. 236 (April 1987)

35. 1974 Occupational Survey, *Mayo Clinic Proceedings*, Vol. 59, (1984)

36. "US Agency Bars Formaldehyde Foam Insulation," *Medical World News*, (March, 15 1982)

37. Acheson, E.D. et al. "Formaldehyde in British Chemical Industry," *Lancet*, (March 1984)

38. *American Cancer Society Journal*. (March 1982)

39. "MMPD in Hair & Fur Dyes," *NIOSH*, 83:105

40. M.J. Prival, et.al.: "Mutagenicity of Benzidine and Benzidine-Congener Dyes and Selected Mono Azo Dyes in a Modified Salmonella Assay," *Mutation Research*, 136 (1984)

41. Graham Sole, and Tom Sorahan, "Fishermen's Dye and Risk of Urotherial Cancer," *Lancet*, (June 29, 1985)

42. *Journal of the American Medical Association*, (June 1983)

43. Mary Wolff, et. al., "Human Tissue Burdens of Halogenated Aromatic Chemicals in Michigan," *Journal of the American Medical Association* Vol. 247 #15, (April 1982)

44. *American Journal of Industrial Medicine* 11:1987

45. Richard Fruncillo, "Clinical Toxicology of PCBs," *American Family Physician*, (1985)

46. *A Consumer's Dictionary of Cosmetic Ingredients*, (New York: Crown Publishers, 1984)

47. *NIOSH* Bulletin #19, 1978

48. *American Journal of Industrial Medicine*, (1982)

49. T.K. Ng, *Medical Journal of Australia*. 1984

50. Daniel Cramer, *Cancer*, (July 1982)

CHAPTER SIX

DIET AND NUTRITION

What you eat every day—from the double cheeseburger and can of diet pop at lunch to the well-marbled, charbroiled steak and glass of wine at dinner—has been the subject of many recent studies which attempt to evaluate the role of diet in the development of cancer

Dr. Peter Greenwald, Director of the National Cancer Institute's Division of Cancer Prevention and Control, writes that over 30 percent of all human cancers are connected to diet, including up to half of all cancers that occur in women and one third of all cancers that occur in men.[1] A bad diet, then, may be second only to tobacco in responsibility for causing cancer. These are American statistics, however; world-wide statistics show a much different picture, reflecting a tremendous variety in dietary and smoking habits.

The components of food which are necessary to support human life are: fats, protein, carbohydrates, fiber, vitamins and minerals. They are dispersed in different food groups—dairy products, meats, fruits, vegetables, grain, and cereals. The amount of each of these food groups consumed varies enormously throughout the world. Excesses and deficiencies in the diets of different countries correspond fairly accurately to differences in cancer rates.

107

The different components of food have widely different roles in initiation and promotion of cancer. For example, deficiency of vitamins and minerals plays a larger role in the initiation phase. Fats and alcohol play a role primarily in the promotion of cancer. Carbohydrates do not appear to have a direct role in causation of cancer, but deficiency of protein is associated with the causation of some cancers. In the following pages, the individual components of the diet are discussed as they relate to cancer.

THE OBESITY-CANCER CONNECTION

Obesity is related to cancer, especially cancer of the uterus, breast, ovaries and prostate. According to Dr. Saul Gusberg of the Mt. Sinai School of Medicine, if you are a female and 21-50 pounds overweight, your risk of cancer of the uterus is three times that of the general population.[2] If you are more than 50 pounds overweight your cancer risk is multiplied nine times. Obese women are two to four times at risk of developing breast cancer compared to non-obese women.[3] Cancer of the ovaries in women and prostate in men are also more prevalent in the obese population.

DID YOU KNOW THAT?

- Approximately 34 million adults in the United States are overweight.[4]

- Approximately 24 percent of men and 27 percent of women in the United States are overweight in a society seized with a "fitness craze."

- Obesity in people is an independent risk factor for chronic diseases like cancer and hypertension.

Since obesity is such a widespread problem in the American population, so are the diseases associated with obesity, including cancer. The main reason for our problems with obesity, quite simply, is that we eat too much. We should not live to eat, but eat to live. High calorie intake combined with a sedentary life-style results in obesity.

Who is obese? The answer is arbitrary, but the Metropolitan Life Insurance Company uses weight levels that are 20 percent or more than normal for certain height and build as their standard for determining obesity.[5] Life insurance companies, along with the medical profession and researchers, have all noted that obese people have higher-than-average rates of breast, colon, ovarian, uterine, and prostate cancers. This rate can be reduced by either lowering the calorie intake in diet or increasing calorie expenditure by exercise. Recent studies have shown that increasing an individual's calorie expenditure by exercise appears to lower the risk of cancer as well as the risks of heart disease. You can literally walk or jog away from cancer.

Exercise for Health

It has been known for a long time that exercise is beneficial for the body in many ways, such as preserving life and desirable qualities into old age. Even though we cannot reverse the aging process, we can avoid or at least defer chronic diseases such as heart disease and cancer. A number of recent studies have confirmed this idea. In a study of 16,936 Harvard Alumni, aged 35 to 74, and followed over the years 1962-78, those alumni that exercised by walking, stair climbing and sports were found to have a significantly lower risk of mortality.[6]

Dr. Rose Frisch at the Harvard School of Public Health conducted another study on over 5,398 physically active females who graduated from college between 1925-1981. Her study showed that non-athletes, when compared to a similar number of physically active females—women who exercised two times a week or played sports like basketball, squash, crew, dance, fencing, field hockey, swimming, tennis, track or volleyball—had a two-and-a-half times higher rate of cancer of the reproductive system and twice the rate of breast cancer. Dr. Frisch felt that regular exercise started early in life appears to reduce the risk of cancer by reducing estrogen secretion.[7]

Dr. Steven Blair and his associates confirmed this finding recently in a study done on close to 15,000 people who were followed for 11 years. In the higher exercise groups, they found lower overall mortality from cardiovascular disease and cancer.[8] People who exercise regularly also appear to have a lower risk of colon cancer.[9]

Let's look at caloric intake next. Analysis of the different food groups shows that fats are a concentrated source of calories and have nine calories per gram; proteins and carbohydrates have four calories per gram; fiber has none.

High Caloric Intake

International studies show that the amounts of fat and fiber people consume varies dramatically from country to country. For example, the major components of an average American's diet are meat and dairy products—which contain a large amount of animal fat—and baked goods made with refined flour. In comparison, the average Japanese diet of raw fish, vegetables and rice is much lower in animal fat and higher in fiber from the large amount of vegetables consumed. Midway between these two extremes is the typical East European diet high in vegetables and dairy products, higher in fiber than the American diet, but somewhere between the Japanese and American diets in fat content.

In each of these three diets, the Japanese, the Eastern European and the Western European/American, fat and fiber ratios differ dramatically. As the dietary fat content increases and fiber content decreases, the rates of certain cancers—colon, breast, and uterus—correspond accordingly.

The daily fat intake of Americans is about twice that of the Japanese. Death from breast cancer in the United States is also more than four times as high as in Japan and death from colon cancer in men is more than three times as high. Nationally, studies of eating patterns show that while the United States may be the land of plenty in the eyes of most other nations, American dietary habits and the resulting health problems leave a great deal to be desired.

Cheeseburgers and well-marbled steaks contribute to a diet that is very high in protein and calories, as well as high in animal fat containing large amounts of cholesterol. The average American's diet is more than 40 percent fat. Fast food diets may contain an even higher percentage of fat. The American Cancer Society recommends no more than 30 percent fat in the diet of the average adult American in its nutrition guidelines. My own belief is that it should be cut to less than 20 percent for any person more than two years of age.

A look at two studies done in the United States on people with eating patterns extremely low in fat and cholesterol intake provide interesting evidence in incriminating fatty foods as causing cancer.

First, consider the Seventh-Day Adventists, a religious group whose practices include a low-fat diet that contains no meat, sparing use of eggs and cheese, and a high consumption of milk for protein. There is little obesity among these people and the rates of prostate cancer in the men have been very low traditionally. 25,000 men in this religious group were compared to a control group in 1960 who regularly ate fattier foods over a 20 year period. The findings: overweight men were more likely to develop prostate cancer and die from this disease than men of average weight.[10]

Female Seventh-Day Adventists were also compared with control groups from the average population. Women from the control group, whose diets included eggs three or more times a week, had a three times higher risk for ovarian cancer than women who ate eggs less than once weekly. Still another ovarian cancer link was found in women whose diets were high in fried foods like bacon or potatoes.[11]

Migrant studies done on different populations provide proof as telling as results from a laboratory. The migration of peoples from a low risk country to a high risk location provides data for an experiment conducted on human beings by nature.[12] Studies done on the health patterns of native Japanese women and those who have migrated to the United States offers more evidence of the problematic connection between a high fat diet and cancer. Native Japanese in general are afflicted with colon, breast and prostate cancer at a lower rate than that of the United States population.

Japanese women living in Japan and eating the traditional Japanese diet low in animal fat, have an extremely low rate of breast cancer. Breast cancer increases dramatically among second generation Japanese women living in America who have adopted a western style of eating. Similarly, colon cancer rates go up in first generation Japanese Americans. Heredity and genetics are not solely responsible for the contrast in these statistics; adopted behavior of eating high fat foods play an important role. The "Westernization" of the Japanese diet has even led to higher rates of colon, breast and prostate cancer in Japan.

How Do Fats Promote Cancer?

Laboratory experiments on animals seem to indicate that cholesterol and other dietary fats are tumor promoters, and studies on rats have shown that high-fat diets make conditions favorable for cancer. Fats have been determined to work in three important ways as cancer promoters.

First, eating a high-fat diet—a concentrated source of calories—stimulates excess secretions of sex hormones, much like putting high octane airplane fuel into the engine of a compact automobile. This leads to higher incidence of cancers of the target organs for sex hormones—the reproductive organs such as breast and uterus in women, and prostate in men. For example, adding calories to the daily diet makes the onset of menarche (menses) occur earlier in pubertal girls, and we know that early age of menarche is a factor associated with breast cancer. We can deduce, therefore, that overfeeding in childhood may render a person over-susceptible to these hormone dependent cancers.

Second, the effect of a high fat diet stimulates bile secretions into the intestines. These bile salts are known tumor promoters in laboratory animals.

The third aspect of fat as a promoter is its relationship to the transit time of fecal material through the intestine. If fecal material travels quickly through the intestines, less cholesterol will be absorbed by the body. A normal length of passage is 24 hours. Some pioneering research has linked the natural chemical processes that occur in the body as it breaks down fat and interacts with certain bile salts and bacteria. Though these bile salts and bacteria are natural and normally present, increased time spent within the gut during this complex interaction can transform these bile salts into carcinogens.

CHOLESTEROL AND CANCER

Animal lab experiments, international and national dietary patterns, and studies on effect of migration of people have all implicated high animal fat in the development of colon cancer. However, the human proof was missing—concrete evidence that would demonstrate the connection between high cholesterol intake in diet and increased cancer risk.

Two 1986 European studies have made the all-important connection that high blood cholesterol in individuals can put them at twice the risk of developing precancerous polyps (adenomas) and cancer of the colon. (High blood cholesterol is generally reflective of high cholesterol in the diet.)

Adenoma (polyps) in the colon are benign tumors found in 20-50 percent of adults over 40 years of age. One interesting observation has been that patients with colonic polyps have been found to have high incidence of coronary artery disease (due to high blood cholesterol). Also, patients with colonic polyps and colon cancer have been found to have high concentration of cholesterol and its metabolites and bile acids in their feces.[13]

Current studies have finally proved that lowering cholesterol can lower incidence of heart disease and colon cancer.

CHOLESTEROL CONTENT OF COMMON FOODS

- Liver or lean beef (6 ozs.):   750 mg.

- One whole egg or one yolk, a six ounce serving of sardines or a can of cooked shrimp: 250 mg.

- Lean beef, lean veal, lean pork, lobster, lean lamb, boiled ham, flounder, dark chicken without skin, or ½ cup of heavy cream: 125 to 175 mg.

- One tablespoon of butter: 35 mg.

- A cup of skim milk, 4 percent fat cottage cheese or low fat yogurt, any amount of peanut butter, pancakes, mayonnaise, one frankfurter, one slice of bread: less than 50 mg.

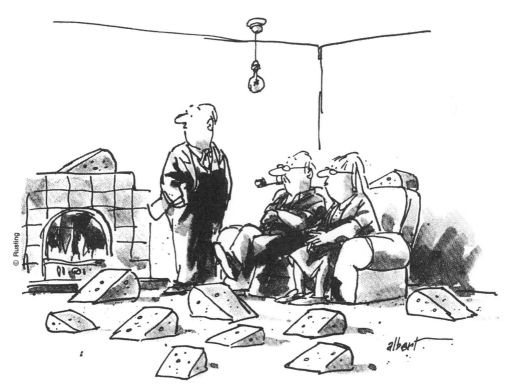

"We haven't got a mousetrap. We're hoping the cholesterol might kill them."

(Reprinted with permission by Punch/Rothco)

These foods all contain *saturated* fats which in turn contain cholesterol. Some saturated fats come from plant or vegetable sources and also are not recommended. Examples are coconut and palm oil, commonly used in non-dairy creamers.

The types of fats that should be used in place of cholesterol-containing fats are *unsaturated* fats—those either solid at room temperature or vegetable oils which are liquid at room temperature. Common sources for unsaturated fats are olive oil, canola oil, corn oil, cottonseed oil, margarine, safflower oil, sunflower oil, soybean oil and peanut oil. Canola oil is probably the best overall. However, in animal experiments, olive oil appears to be devoid of promoting effects of breast cancer and colon cancer similar to fish oils.

Current recommendations about dietary fat intake are that fats should not contribute more than 20 percent of the total calorie intake. Following this guideline could reduce the risk of breast and colon cancer by as much as 80 percent. This recommendation is especially important for those at high risk for colon cancer (with polyps) or breast cancer (with cystic breast disease).

The conditions for promoting cancer are cumulative, built up over years of dietary habits and patterns. What can we do to make changes in lifelong conditions? One way is by eating a diet that is lower in animal fats. A second is by interfering with the absorption of cholesterol in these fats by adding fiber.

FIBER

Hippocrates, the father of medicine, advised use of bran in the 5th century. Over the last few years much attention has been given to the miraculous effects of fiber upon the human digestive system. Body and exercise gurus like Richard Simmons and Jane Fonda have been quick to laud its importance for weight control to the body-conscious public.

What is fiber, and what is its relationship to cancer? Fiber is the partially indigestible carbohydrate material that is abundant in fruits, vegetables, grains and cereals.

A high fiber diet has been associated with lower rates of colon cancer in Africa and Asia. Study of the fiber content of diets in western countries such as Finland shows a diet high in both animal fats and fiber. Accordingly, Finland has low instances of colon cancer. Similarly in Greece, people eat lots of fiber and cook with olive oil, creating correspondingly low rates of colon cancer.

The average American diet contains only 10-30 grams of fiber compared to the African diet's 90 grams.[14] According to the American Cancer Society, fiber in the American diet should be increased to 50-60 grams daily. This can be done by consuming high fiber foods, processed foods containing fiber or fiber preparations available in the drug stores. The best way to increase your fiber is to eat high fiber foods which have the additional value of large amounts of vitamins and mineral. Natural foods are clearly preferable to fiber supplements or fiber enriched cereals. Nonetheless, although the value of fiber supplements has not been proven, they have been found helpful in lowering cholesterol.

HIGH FIBER FOODS

FRUITS: oranges, grapefruits, pineapples, apples, bananas, peaches, pears, apricots, berries, cantaloupes, papayas, prunes, raisins, and plums. Unstrained fruit juices.

VEGETABLES: carrots, winter squash, turnips, tomatoes, cabbage, cauliflower, Brussels sprouts, potatoes, sweet potatoes, broccoli, corn, parsnips, kale, spinach, celery, green beans, yams, and greens.

WHOLE WHEAT: whole wheat, rye, oatmeal, pumpernickel, bran and corn breads; whole grain crackers; whole wheat pasta; whole wheat breakfast cereals like oatmeal, shredded wheat and raisin bran.

GRAINS: brown rice, barley, popcorn, etc.

DRIED BEANS: black, kidney, garbanzo, pinto, navy, white, lima, lentils, black eye peas, and split peas.

DRIED FRUITS: apricots, prunes, figs, peaches, and dates.

NUTS AND SEEDS: all types.

Other foods made with whole grain flours like waffles, pancakes, pasta and taco shells are available, too.

How Fiber Works

Even though fiber is not digestible, it is a necessary component in a well-balanced diet, mainly because it adds bulk and also increases the amount of water in the stool. This shortens transit time of the stool through the intestines. British researcher Dennis Burkitt published a landmark study in 1972 demonstrating the connection of fiber to efficient human excretion. He showed that in diets containing high fiber, stool bulk was 400 G/d, or nearly twice the average of a person on an American diet consisting of mainly refined carbohydrates.[15]

The transit time becomes much more efficient if large amounts of fiber are eaten in the diet. The longer the stool remains in the intestines, the longer time potential carcinogens in the stool have to wreak havoc on the intestinal lining. The extra water held by fiber in the stool can also "dilute" potential carcinogens. In addition, fiber and water can alter the bacteria which is normally present in the intestines (discussed in the section on cholesterol).

Recent studies on patients with high blood cholesterol have shown that the addition of regular amounts of commercial fiber preparations commonly used as bulk laxatives decrease the cholesterol in these patients by 10-15 percent.[16]

In summary, the role of fiber in preventing cancer is a secondary one: it dilutes the cholesterol and bile salts in the gut, interfering with their absorption into the body, and removing them from the body efficiently.

THE ANTICANCER POWER OF VITAMINS

The search for agents to prevent cancer goes on. We have developed a "quick fix" mentality, and people in general would prefer a *prescription* over *proscription*. The search for "prescriptions" leads many of us to vitamins.

There are 14 vitamins essential to the human diet. Of these, vitamins are generally grouped into two categories according to their solubility: fat or water. For example, vitamins B and C are water soluble; if you take them in an excess quantity they will be filtered out of the body through the urine. On the other hand, vitamins A, D, E, and K are fat soluble and are stored in the liver and fatty tissues of the body. They eliminate rather slowly from the body, so toxicity and adverse reactions from taking megadoses have been known to occur.

Consumption Trends

The popularity of vitamins continues to rise, and many Americans take a daily vitamin supplement. However, the average American eats 1,425 pounds of food a year and each of the three essential vitamins, A, C, and E, is readily available from a well balanced diet.

Vitamins A, C, and E have been receiving special attention from researchers as they look for deeper clues and explanations for cancer prevention. The special link between these three vitamins is that they are all anti-oxidants, meaning that they interfere with the damage done by chemical carcinogens to genetic material such as DNA.

In the two stages of cancer formation, initiation and promotion, it has been found that vitamins inhibit only the promotional stage. They also appear to stimulate the immune system.

Vitamin A and Beta-Carotene

In 1925, Dr. Y. Fujimaki found that mice fed a vitamin A deficient diet developed stomach cancer at a higher rate than mice fed on a normal diet containing vitamin A. This early experiment showed the protective effect of vitamin A against cancer.

In the subsequent decades, the effect of vitamin A was studied extensively in laboratory experiments. The results proved not only that a vitamin A deficiency could increase the risk of lung and bladder cancer in mice, but also that natural compounds with vitamin A were able to prevent breast, skin and bladder cancer. These compounds, such as beta-carotene and synthetic derivatives of vitamin A called retinoids, were shown to suppress the malignant behavior of the cultured cells in the laboratory when transformed by chemicals, radiation and viruses. But the doses of the vitamin A compounds used were ten to 20 times higher than the normal recommended daily allowance for humans.

Because vitamin A compounds have shown such a powerful anti-cancer effect in animals, population studies have been done on humans to examine the dosage of vitamin A and beta-carotene (B-carotene) and subsequent risk of cancer. A number of questionnaire studies have been done by charting the intake of foods containing vitamin A and beta-carotene, such as fruits and vegetables. In 1975, Erik Bjelke, a professor of Hygiene at the University of Bergen in Norway, asked 8,278 men what they ate. Following these men for five years, he determined that the incidence of cancer was four and a half times higher in those with a low vitamin A diet.[17]

Similarly in a Hawaiian study, Dr. Ward Hinds and his associates compared a survey of 364 cancer patients with 627 people of general population. They found that there was twice an increased risk of lung cancer in men associated with low vitamin A and beta-carotene consumption.[18] And at the State University of New York at Buffalo, Dr. Tim Byers found that beta-carotene intake in fruits was associated with a lower risk of lung cancer.

Vitamin A intake not only has been studied in relation to lung cancer, but to other cancers as well. A low vitamin A intake may increase the risk of laryngeal cancer by two times[19] and the risk of stomach cancer by two times.[20]

Increased beta-carotene intake has shown a lower incidence of oral, throat, esophageal, stomach, bladder and cervical cancers. This clearly indicates the protective effect of beta-carotene against many epithelial cancers. (Epithelial cells line the skin, gastrointestinal tract, bronchial tubes in the lungs, bladder and the cervix of the uterus.)

Role in Precancerous Conditions

Vitamin A appears to suppress the promotional phase of carcinogenesis. It has shown its effectiveness against cancer in many precancerous situations.

One of the synthetic vitamin A derivatives (a retinoid) called Transretinoic Acid (TRA) was used as a cervical cap to deliver the retinoids locally for cervical dysplasia, a precancerous condition of the cervix. According to a University of Arizona team headed by Dr. Frank Meyskenes Jr., the cervical dysplasia completely disappeared in half of the patients after this treatment.

A similar success has been achieved with retinoid treatment for laryngeal papillomas in children, which is a warty growth on vocal nodules due to HPV (human papilloma virus) infection transmitted to the baby from the mother at the time of birth.

Oral leukoplakias are white plaques in the lining of the mouth that develop in response to local irritation. These were recognized as precancerous as early as 1870 by Dr. James Paget, who labelled them "smokers patch." Ten to 12 percent of these patches will become cancerous over a period of one to twenty years.[21] This sequence of events—leukoplakia to cancer—has been seen in laboratory experiments with hamsters and also in human beings. Retinoic acid successfully regressed these patches, and similar results were obtained with beta-carotene and vitamin E. All of the agents work similarly on affecting the genetic material as antioxidants, and through boosting the immune system. Currently a mouth wash containing retinoids is being developed at Yale University for treatment of leukoplakia.

Other precancerous conditions that are being conquered by the retinoids are:

- Preleukemias (myelodysplastic syndrome),[22]

- Dysplastic nevi: abnormal moles that turn into malignant melanoma,

- Keratoacanthoma: a skin cancer,

- Pulmonary metaplasia: abnormal changes in the lining of the bronchial tubes in the lungs of smokers.

Advanced Cancers

A lymphatic cancer of the skin called mycosis fungoides has been treated with retinoids at the University of Arizona. Out of 18 patients, nine had partial remission, two had minor response, and two others experienced total remission lasting several years. This "home run" was scored by use of retinoic acid.[23]

SOURCES OF VITAMIN A AND BETA-CAROTENE (B-CAROTENE)

Vitamin A, by itself, is rare in foods from animal sources, except in cod liver oil. It is found primarily in plant sources in the form of "Pro Vit A" beta-carotene. Some examples of these sources of beta-carotene are: salads, green beans, asparagus, spinach, broccoli, yellow fruits and vegetables such as apricots, peaches, tomatoes, carrots, squash, white and sweet potatoes. Animal sources of vitamin A are mainly dairy products, fish and liver.

Vitamin B

The members of the vitamin B family have not been linked to cancer to date. Nonetheless, the B vitamin folic acid is a subject of many studies underway in the area of chemoprevention trials by the National Cancer Institute. Folic acid has been found to reduce chances of chromosomal breaks that may lead to cancer and may be used as a protective agent. Vitamin B, like vitamin C, should be taken after a large meal because it is water soluble.

Vitamin C

Vitamin C has a very important role in the growth and maintenance of connective tissues of the body. It has received more instant recognizability than the 13 other vitamins necessary to human functions and good health, mainly because Dr. Linus Pauling preached about the virtue of orange juice as a powerful preventative for colds.

In late 1960, new evidence led to thinking that vitamin C increased the resistance to the development of cancer in a number of ways. By enhancing the immune system, vitamin C increased the body's ability to cope with formation of and the spread of cancers. It could also prevent the conversion of dietary nitrites into nitrosamines, the deadly cancer-causing chemicals, in the stomach.

In laboratory experiments on hamster lung tissues, vitamin C appears to reduce the cancer-causing effect of tobacco and marijuana by preventing the derangements in cell division. Dr. Sylvia Wassertheil-Smoller and associates deduced from these findings that vitamin C might have similar results in humans, reducing the carcinogenic effects of tobacco smoke in lung cancer.[24]

By inhibiting the formation of some cancer-causing chemicals like nitrosamines from nitrites in the diet, vitamin C lowers the risk of cancers of the esophagus and stomach. In 1970, Dr. Pauling and Dr. E. Cameron, after working with 128 terminally ill patients at Vale of Leven

Hospital in Scotland, observed that megadoses of vitamin C enhanced the immune system and had a positive survival effect on patients suffering from cancer.[25] The use of vitamin C has also produced a reduction in risk of secondary cancers in patients with cancers of the cervix, mouth, esophagus, stomach and larynx.[26]

According to the Health and Nutrition Examination Survey, about 35 percent of women aged 25-44 in the United States have daily vitamin C intakes of 30 mg. and 68 percent have intakes below 88 mg.[27]

Vitamin C-Rich Foods and Their Use

Fruits: Oranges and other citrus fruits, such as grapefruits, lemons, oranges, and pineapples; pears and cantaloupe.

Vegetables: broccoli, Brussels sprouts, cabbage, cauliflower, tomatoes, paprika, bell peppers, salad greens.

Vitamin C is a very sensitive vitamin, easily destroyed by cooking, mincing, air exposure or contact with copper utensils. It should be eaten with every meal, since it is water soluble and is filtered out of the body quickly.

What a happy coincidence that we make such partnerships as ham with pineapple, bacon with orange juice, and nitrate cured corn beef with vitamin C rich cabbage, pastrami, and cole slaw! In these combinations, the nitrosamines of bacon, ham, and corn beef are being neutralized by the vitamin C rich foods.

Vitamin D

The relationship of vitamin D to cancer is not yet known, but since it promotes the absorption of calcium from the gut, taking normal recommended amounts can cause no harm.

Vitamin E

Like vitamin C, vitamin E is an anti-oxidant, which means it "rust proofs" our cell walls.[28] Vitamin E has been found to be an effective preventative against lung cancer in some animal studies and in one human study, confirmed by Dr. Paul Knekt and associates from Finland.[29] They showed that subjects with higher blood levels of vitamin E were at a lower risk for cancer in general. In the United States, vitamin E is being studied for its preventive effects by the National Cancer Institute in Chemoprevention Trials. Researcher Garry Duthie, of Scotland, found in a study that vitamin E seems to shield the cells of the bronchial tubes from damage caused by cigarette smoke.[30]

SOURCES OF VITAMIN E

Vitamin E has been found in almonds, sunflower seeds, sesame seeds, whole grain cereals, other vegetable oils like canola, soya bean and corn oils, and eggs.

MINERALS IN THE DIET

Minerals in the diet have not been the subject of much conclusive testing in their relationship to cancer. Studies of populations over a period of time are usually concerned with exposures to minerals from the workplace environment rather than from the diet. Nonetheless, some laboratory tests have been conducted on some twenty trace elements and minerals. When added to the drinking water of rats, arsenic, cadmium, lead, zinc, calcium, selenium and iodine appeared to show some evidence of a relationship to cancer. Cadmium compounds are routinely mutagenic to cells cultured in the laboratory (see Chapter Five on chemicals, for a discussion of arsenic). Lead, when inhaled even indirectly or consumed in drinking water and in food, does correlate with stomach, intestinal, ovarian and renal cancers.

Calcium

There have been a number of reports that have linked an insufficient intake of calcium to osteoporosis, hypertension and, more recently, to cancer. Population studies have shown that subjects with higher intake of calcium (in milk) show a lower incidence of colon cancer. The Finnish diet is high in calcium and Finns have lower rates of colon cancer—despite a high dietary fat intake. Calcium apparently has the ability to bind bowel irritants such as fatty acids and bile salts, by making insoluble calcium soaps. This process facilitates the prompt excretion of cancer-causing agents.[31]

In experiments on animals, the addition of calcium to the diet has been linked with a lower incidence of colon, breast and stomach cancers. Several studies are underway in this country under the auspices of the National Cancer Institute; supplemental calcium is being given to high risk groups such as potential colon cancer victims with the hereditary condition of familial polyps.

Drinking two to three glasses of skim milk fortified with vitamin B daily is a safe bet as a preventative against colon cancer—possibly reducing the risk of this cancer three-fold, according to a study by Dr. Cedric Garland of the University of California.

121

Selenium

Selenium was first recognized to be an essential mineral in the 1950s. It is found in seafood and organ meats and to a lesser extent in whole grain cereals, meat and poultry, and appears to offer some protection against the formation of cancer. The right amount in the diet seems to do the trick, which is about 50-200 mg. a day.[32] Low levels of dietary selenium are common among populations with an increased incidence of skin, lung and colon cancers. Cancer patients themselves often show decreased levels of selenium in their blood. Three studies done in this area—two in Finland and one in the United States—have shown three times increased risk of lung cancer with a lower intake of selenium.

Too much selenium, however, can be toxic. Selenium added to the drinking water could have a preventative effect against tumors from chemical carcinogens, but large doses of selenium have not been shown to be more effective than average doses of it. Selenium is also being studied by the National Cancer Institute in chemoprevention trials in the United States and China. At present, a selenium supplement is not recommended for the general population. Some nursing home patients or others not eating a well-balanced diet can be supplemented with selenium-rich yeast preparations.

Zinc

The relationship of zinc to cancer and the immune system is covered in Chapter Eight on Contagious Cancers and the Immune System.

ALCOHOL AND CANCER

Alcohol has probably been around since prehistoric times. Its use has been seen throughout recorded human history: Egyptian wall paintings depict beer and wine making; Homer tells of the intoxication of the Cyclops in the Odyssey; and Biblical stories describe the use of mead, a drink made by the fermentation of honey and water.

Alcohol is consumed in great quantities throughout the world—except in countries like Saudi Arabia where its use has been prohibited by law. In the United States, alcohol is a popular over-the-counter tranquilizer and it can be purchased easily. About two-thirds of the United States population drink alcoholic beverages. Alcohol makes up nearly 25 percent of the caloric intake of the average adult American's diet. The reasons for alcohol consumption are not hard to understand; "drinking" has become associated with enhanced social skills and leisure activities.

Unfortunately, alcohol consumption appears to be increasing, especially among young adults. It rose 21 percent during the 1960s, 10.3 percent during the 1970s, reached a plateau in 1980, and declined somewhat after 1984. The 1984 consumption rate was estimated to be about 2.65 gallons of absolutely pure alcohol for United States residents over 14 years of age. According to recent statistics, approximately 10.6 million adults in the United States are classified as alcoholics, 7.3 million are alcohol abusers, and 4.6 million teenagers 14 to 17 years of age are problem drinkers.[33] These numbers contribute to many social and marital problems, as well as other hazards. Half of the total number of automobile accidents, one-third of all small aircraft crashes and two-thirds of all violent crimes are alcohol related.

Alcohol abuse also causes various health problems such as pancreatitis, nutritional deficiencies, cancers, fetal alcohol syndrome, and cirrhosis of the liver. Alcohol can be an important cause of malnutrition in alcoholics; they often get more than half of their calories from alcohol, empty calories lacking the essential nutrients. The damage done to society by alcohol comes to *100,000 deaths* and economic costs of *120 billion dollars annually*—an expensive addiction.[34]

Out of all the medical problems associated with alcohol use, cancer is one of the most serious. A Boston surgeon in 1837 was the first to make the connection between alcohol and cancer in a patient who had cancer of the tongue, chewed tobacco, and was generated by "long and ardent use of spirits." It is estimated that about three percent of all cancers are caused by alcohol.

The Chemistry of a Drink

What is "a drink?" A drink is defined as one ounce of whiskey, gin or any other distilled liquor which is 85 proof (42.5 percent alcohol)—approximately an eighth of a measuring cup.

What we drink for pleasure and leisure is not pure alcohol. Many brews contain powerful carcinogenic chemicals, some of which are contaminants like nitrosamines, pesticide residues such as arsenic, fuel oils containing tar carcinogenic compounds, and dyes. Urethane, often used as a fermentation product, is a powerful chemical and carcinogenic. Many other additives, classified as trade secrets, are used to flavor and enhance the taste of the drink. Beer and wine are strained through asbestos filters, contaminating the beverage with millions of asbestos fibers per liter. There is no standard mode of preparation for homemade varieties, so the possibility of contaminants there is unlimited.

Alcohol also acts as an excellent solvent, dissolving many other carcinogenic chemicals and facilitating their entry into the different cells of the body. It does this by promoting intimate contact between carcinogenic agents and the epithelium (lining of the gut).[35]

Effects on the Body

Alcohol is a toxic compound. It is associated with many medical problems like cirrhosis of the liver, pancreatitis, stomach ulcers, heart failure, toxicity of the immune system and increased susceptibility to infections. According to research done by Dr. Bruce A. Buehler at the University of Nebraska Medical Center, consumption of alcohol during pregnancy can cause birth defects in the fetus and increased risk of cancer in newborns. Compared to mothers who do not consume alcohol during pregnancy, the risk of cancer in their babies is three times greater for those that do. The main areas where cancers appear in these babies are in the kidneys and spinal cord. As we know from our experience with DES (Diethylstilbestrol), drugs are able to cross the placental barrier and cause cancer in the fetus. Therefore, if a mother drinks during pregnancy, she is very likely predisposing her child to an increased risk of cancer in ten to twenty years.[36]

Cancer Risk From Alcohol

As mentioned earlier, three percent of the total cancer occurrence in humans is caused by alcohol. Alcohol is associated with many cancers, including mouth and tongue cancer. It also plays an important role in liver cancer. Even alcohol-containing mouth-washes have been incriminated; two studies done on women who use large amounts of mouth-washes show an increased rate of oral cancer.[37]

The high rates of laryngeal, esophageal, stomach and colo-rectal cancer, especially rectal cancer, have been linked with beer. Alcohol consumption has also been linked to bladder cancer.[38]

Alcohol and Lung Cancer

Alcohol has also been associated with increasing the risk of lung cancer. Many studies done on human beings and in laboratory experiments have shown that alcohol promotes favorable conditions for cancer from tobacco.[39] The combination of drinking and smoking presents a case of double jeopardy. Consuming alcohol in bars and restaurants where second-hand smoke is present is also risky.

Alcohol and Breast Cancer

A number of studies have shown a relationship between alcohol and breast cancer. Dr. Robert A. Hiatt and the late Dr. Richard D. Bawol studied 96,595 female members of Kaiser-Permanente Health plan of Northern California between 1964 and 1972. The women who reported consuming an average of three or more drinks a day had a 40 percent higher risk of breast cancer.[40] Similarly, an increased risk of breast cancer in a study of 89,538 women between the ages of 34 and 59 was reported by Dr. W.C. Willett and associates.[41] They found that women using 15 gms. of alcohol or more per day were at 2.5 times the risk of breast cancer as compared to non-drinkers.

What to do About Alcohol?

Alcohol is a highly addictive drug. Addiction is promoted by carefully planned commercials for beer and wine portraying glamorous and popular personalities. Many of the same types of images are seen in cigarette advertisements. As a result, bars have become a prominent setting for American dating and mating rituals, and a business lunch often includes white wine or a cocktail. The ads promoting these customs are worth 1.2 billion dollars annually.[42]

What can be done? Alcohol consumption appears to be one of those social practices that will probably always be with us in western society. It would be hard to imagine many of life's important celebrations without it. Some people feel alcohol has some beneficial qualities, such as having a tranquilizing effect. French and Italians have always considered it an important part of their cuisine as an aid to digestion. Moderation is probably the key, but moderate drinking can vary enormously from individual to individual because of differences in body weight and hereditary tolerance. As an old proverb goes: "Who is an alcoholic? I guess he who drinks one drink more than me!"

Public outcry against alcohol abuse has increased and has led to the formation of groups which deal with alcohol related problems. SMART (Stop Marketing Alcohol on Radio and TV) and MADD (Mothers Against Drunk Driving) are two groups that are concerned with consequences of alcohol on health and life. Legislative steps that can be taken would be to increase the price of alcohol, increase taxation on alcohol and require the use of labels warning about effects and additives. Legislators could demand better education in the schools and colleges about the detrimental effects of alcohol.

COFFEE — WHAT'S BREWING?

Called by many names—kophe, kava, gahveh, etc.—coffee is still the world's favorite beverage. It was first discovered in the mountains of Ethiopia in the 10th century.

125

DID YOU KNOW THAT?

- The average American drinks 560 cups of coffee per year, down from 1,000 cups in 1946. Soft drink consumption has filled that gap.
- 30 percent of the population drinks a decaffeinated brand of coffee.
- The majority of Americans (72 percent) drink coffee for the taste of it. Forty-two percent drink it to "get them going" in the morning.

What, exactly, is brewing in that cup of coffee? This question has been the subject of much scientific study.

Tar compounds containing polycyclic hydrocarbons (PAH) are produced in coffee as the coffee bean ripens and in the roasting process. These compounds are known carcinogens. Caffeine by itself is a weak mutagen that can enhance the breaks in the chromosomes at fragile sites and inhibit DNA repair during the natural cell division—which may lead to cancer. Individual solvents that are used in processing decaffeinated coffee, such as methylene chloride, are suspected to be human carcinogens.

Recent studies have linked patients suffering from bladder, pancreatic, and colo-rectal cancer with heavy coffee intake. Dr. Brian McMahon and his associates caused quite an uproar when they published a study reporting that coffee drinkers are at almost twice the risk of developing pancreatic cancer as compared to non-drinkers, and at more than two-and-a-half times the risk if they drink three or more cups of coffee daily.[43] These findings were substantiated by another study by Dr. Lorraine Marrett which reported that coffee drinkers increase their risk of bladder cancer one-and-a-half times if they drink seven cups a day.[44]

There seems to be yet another connection between coffee intake, high saturated fat intake and tumor formation in laboratory rats. Dr. J.P. Minton of the American Cancer Society found that tumors did not develop as quickly in these rats if they were fed caffeine without saturated fat.[45]

THE DEADLY NITROSAMINES

Nitrosamines are one of the most potent animal carcinogens known, causing nearly all types of cancer in laboratory animals. They were first discovered to be animal carcinogens in 1956 by Drs. P.N. McGee and J. M. Barnes when they caused liver cancer in laboratory rats.[46] In humans they are highly suspected of being carcinogens in esophageal and stomach cancers, and brain tumors. We are exposed to them from

126

many sources; cigarette smoke, our diet, air and water pollution from nitrates in fertilizers, as well as our own digestive functions.

From time immemorial, nitrates and nitrites such as saltpeter have been used to cure poultry, bacon, sausages, hot dogs and lunch meats, cheese, and fish, mainly to prevent growth of bacteria that cause botulism (food poisoning). Botulism no longer presents the threat it once did because of refrigeration, but nitrates have taken on a more cosmetic function and are often used to give meat a red, fresh look to improve sales.

Fresh vegetables often contain detectable levels of nitrates from the pesticides and fertilizers used in their cultivation. These nitrates and nitrites stored within the food can become converted by the body's own digestive processes into nitrosamines. In some products, such as grilled or fried bacon, these nitrosamines have already formed before the digestive interaction occurs.

We are also exposed to nitrosamines that are in the air from tobacco smoke, industrial pollution and auto exhaust fumes. Drinking water is another source for nitrosamines. Water sources are polluted by industrial discharges and rainwater runoffs on farms, carrying the fertilizer and pesticide residues to lakes and rivers. Pickled vegetables and the dried, salted fish popular in oriental diets are also full of these dangerous compounds.

It appears that vitamin C and vitamin E can interfere with the formation of nitrosamine, and vitamin C is now routinely added to cured bacon sold for public consumption.[47]

AFLATOXINS

Aflatoxins are one of the most potent carcinogens in the diet in microgram quantities. They were first discovered in 1960, when hatchery-reared rainbow trout were found to have a small epidemic of liver cancer after being fed cottonseed oil contaminated with aflatoxin.[48] We now know that aflatoxins are not just one compound but a group of highly toxic compounds found in moldy foods. The foods are contaminated when they are harvested and/or stored, and include peanuts, corn, maize, cottonseed, and other tree nuts, and to some extent other foods. They have been linked to increases in esophageal and liver cancers. High incidence of liver cancers have been reported in African countries and in Asia, where contaminated foods are a usual feature of the diet. These aflatoxins cause suppression of the immune system, allowing infections to rage uncontrolled. For example, the high rate of aflatoxin-contaminated foods are mostly in those areas of the world, namely Africa and Asian countries, where there is a high carriage rate of hepatitis B virus and liver cancer.

CHARCOAL BROILING AND BARBECUING

Charcoal broiling is an all-American culinary pastime. Cancer-causing substances called polycyclic hydrocarbons (PAH) are formed when wood, paper or charcoal are burned and, just as in the case of tobacco smoke, are carried through to the food by smoke and flames.

What is the least carcinogenic way to barbecue foods? By cooking in a conventional oven under the flames. But if barbecue cookery is your summertime recreation, a few suggestions will minimize these risks:

- Cover the charcoal coals with foil to prevent foods from being exposed to smoke;

- Cook meats as far away from the coals as possible; and,

- Remove the skin from chicken after charbroiling.

Microwave cooking also prevents the formation of cancer causing chemicals.

FERMENTED FOODS (Urethane)

Ethylcarbamate or urethane is a product found in wines as a result of fermentation, and it is due to a chemical called diethylpolycarbonate used as a sterilizer in making wines. Small amounts of urethane are also found naturally in wines, beers, yogurt and bread.

Urethane is not known to cause cancer in human beings but has been found to cause cancers in laboratory animals.

BRACKEN FERN

Bracken fern is a plant which is distributed differently around the world and grows wild in some countries. In Japan, it is consumed as food. However, Bracken fern is suspected to cause bladder and esophageal cancer in laboratory animals and human beings. A recent report in the *Medical Tribune* described the carcinogenic poisons released by Bracken fern plants, and a warning was issued to backpackers and hitch-hikers to stay away from these plants, or to at least wear a mask if they were in an area where they would be exposed.[49]

FOOD ADDITIVES: A RAPIDLY GROWING SHOPPING LIST

Acids, alkalies, buffers and neutralizers, moisture content controllers, coloring agents, flavorings, physiologic activity controls; bleaching and maturing agents, bread improvers, processing aids, nutrition supplements: these are among the 2,700 food additives currently used in processing, packaging, and storing food for the market place.[50] Many are manmade chemicals, and nearly everyone—consumers, environmentalists, and manufacturers—worries about their potential as carcinogens.

Since the Food, Drug and Cosmetic Act of 1938, the United States Government has attempted to pass food regulations that would protect the consumer and encourage food manufacturers to set responsible testing standards and controls.

1958 was an important year to remember regarding the United States Government's role as a regulator of food additives. First, upon sifting through the recommendations from an assembled panel of 200 experts, the United States Congress established the GRAS List (Generally Recommended As Safe) of additives for foods. That year Congress also amended the Food, Drug and Cosmetic Act of 1938 with the Delaney Clause, an amendment which prohibits the use of food additives that cause cancer in animals and humans.

As the food industry expanded, it became obvious that the initial GRAS list was not specific enough. More categories were added, but not before the Delaney Clause got into difficulty: the year was 1977, and the issue was saccharin.

Artificial Sweeteners

Americans like sweets. Of the 1,425 pounds of food the average American consumes each year, about 126 pounds are sugar, and an additional 15.8 pounds are in foods containing sugar substitutes—saccharin and aspartame—largely in soft drinks. The consumption of beverages in general had increased from 114 gallons per person in 1962 to 133 gallons in 1982; in the same period, soft drink consumption increased from 16 gallons per person to 39.5. The soft drink market continues to rise.[51]

Saccharin, the oldest of the sugar substitutes, was developed in 1879 as a derivative of petroleum. It underwent some changes in the original formula to eliminate the bitter aftertaste.

Saccharin versus Cyclamates

Saccharin became a highly successful product, helped by a lax interpretation of the law and good timing. First, the food additive laws require proof of safety and efficacy, not of benefit. Thus, a sweetener must sweeten food, but it does not need to have any useful purpose beyond that. Saccharin does that, as it is about 300 times sweeter than sugar (sucrose) on a measuring scale of sweetness levels. Besides, the nation became more diet and health conscious, and the diet pop market burgeoned.

At first, saccharin was used in combination with cyclamates, but by 1969, cyclamates were found to cause bladder cancer in laboratory tests on rats and were taken off the market in the United States and in Great Britain. Cyclamates are widely used in Canada where saccharin is banned. These and further studies on cyclamates are now considered inconclusive, and the product is used widely in nearly every other country in the world. It may reappear in our marketplace in the near future.

With the ban on cyclamate, saccharin had the diet pop market all to itself. By 1976, seven million pounds of saccharin was being used in foods, table top sweeteners, mouthwash, toothpaste, and prescription drugs for pediatric use. About 14 percent of the consumers are estimated to be teenagers. Contrary to popular belief, only a third of all diabetics in the United States use saccharin regularly.

Saccharin has been tested exhaustively over the past 40 years on laboratory animals and on human beings. Some studies have been sponsored by industry, some by government. Saccharin has been recognized as a low potency carcinogen and a tumor promoter in laboratory rats.[52] It has been banned in Canada because of a study conducted by the Canadian Health Protection Branch, which found that laboratory rats fed saccharin developed cancer in 1977.

Human studies, particularly for carcinogens, are difficult to conduct properly. First of all, cancer has a long latency period (30-40 years), and enough time needs to elapse between exposure and disease. Second, a large enough sampling of exposed and unexposed individuals has to be available. Third, there is a certain synergism that takes place when two or three chemicals are taken into the body at the same time, and the results are easily altered by the introduction of another additive. The most important study on saccharin was done by the Wisconsin Alumni Research Foundation in 1972, known as the WARF Study. It suggested a link between saccharin and bladder cancer in rats as cited in the 1975 *National Academy of Sciences* Report. A 1976 study in the *Journal of Food Science* cites a study on rats which were given one additive and stayed healthy, then became sick after two additives were introduced at the same time in their diets. This example just hints at the complexity of the problems of attempting to study food additives.[53]

Two Canadian studies greatly contributed to the study of saccharin. One was conducted on laboratory rats who developed bladder cancer at very high rates after being fed the equivalent of 800 cans of diet soda daily. The second, published in the British medical magazine *Lancet*, cited men who were diagnosed as having bladder cancer in three

Canadian provinces. They were matched against neighborhood controls, and it was found that men who had used saccharin had a 65 percent greater chance of developing bladder cancer than those in the control group. Risk increased with duration and amount of use.

The FDA released the information from the rat studies in a newsletter. It did not cite its own testing programs on saccharin, but indicated that extreme testing, such as that done in the Canadian tests, was required by the terms of the Delaney Amendment. The one decisive action that came out of the controversy was that all saccharin-enhanced products were required to carry a warning label of cancer in laboratory rats.

Aspartame (NutraSweet)

American ingenuity once again saved the day by creating a new sweetening agent, called aspartame and commonly known as Nutra-Sweet. However, aspartame brought with it a new set of worries. It was first developed in laboratories in the late 1960s, and by 1974, this new product had entered the artificial sweetener scene and was approved for foods but not for soft drinks. It was approved for use in soda pop in 1983. Technically, aspartame is not an artificial sweetener but a combination of two amino acids (phenylalanine and aspartic acid), constituents of proteins found in meat, milk, and eggs. These just happen to taste sweet when placed in the right combination.

Aspartame (NutraSweet) now dominates the marketplace. In 1985, more than 70 products contained it, yielding sales of four billion dollars. About 180 times sweeter than sugar, aspartame contains one-tenth the calories. But again, the full story on the safety of aspartame is not in yet. So far, the safety studies done by the manufacturer showing a risk of brain tumors in rats have been criticized by Congress as selective and outdated.[54] Legislation has been introduced to have the additive tested by an independent agency rather than the manufacturer.

One thing we do know about aspartame is that it cannot be used in cooking because it is affected by temperatures over 100° F. At this point, aspartame breaks down and changes to methanol or wood alcohol, which can be harmful to fetal brain development and cause eye problems. Even brain tumors and dizziness have been linked to use of aspartame.

Food Colors and Dyes

Natural plant dyes were the cornerstone of the food coloring industry until the latter part of the 19th century when a young English

YOUR CHOICE OF COLORS

The synthetic food dyes listed here have been approved by the FDA for use in foods.

DYE COLOR*	USED IN	CONCERNS
Red no. 40 *2.7 million*	Soda, candy, desserts, pastry, sausage	Lymphomas found in one animal test; findings dismissed by FDA as insignificant
Red no. 3 *253,000*	Cherries, candy, baked goods	Thyroid tumors in male rats; panel debating findings; suit by Public Citizen on appeal
Yellow no. 6 *1.6 million*	Beverages, sausage, baked goods, candy, gelatin	Allergies in some people; kidney tumors in one animal test; FDA concluded tumors not associated with dye
Yellow no. 5 *1.5 million*	Desserts, candy, baked goods	Allergies, mostly in aspirin-sensitive people
Green no. 3 *5,000*	Candy, beverages	Bladder tumors in one animal test; FDA found tumors not associated with dye
Blue no. 1 *217,000*	Beverages, candy, baked goods	Kidney tumors in male mice; findings deemed insignificant by FDA
Blue no. 2 *85,000*	Beverages, candy	Brain tumors in one animal test; FDA dismissed link to dye; suit by Public Citizen on appeal

Pounds used in 1986; actual colors are shown.

By Mary James (Reprinted from *Hippocrates - The Magazine of Health & Medicine,* ©1987 Hippocrates Partners)

chemistry student, William Henry Perkin, discovered that dyes could be made out of coal tars which resisted fading from sunlight and did not come out in the wash water.

In 1906, the United States Congress approved the registration of seven of these coal-tar based colors for use as additives to food. The list of approved colors grew. By 1938, Congress required that manufacturers test and register each new color, but many colors were registered provisionally. At the time, in the early 20th century, consumers and government regulators were far more worried about contamination from bacteria in food than they were about cancer.

Coal tar products have become the largest single class of F. D. & C. (Food, Drug and Cosmetic) colors, used in everything from beverages to food, chewing gum, cosmetics, textiles and paints. It is estimated that from 1950 to 1984 the consumption of food colors tripled. The F.D.A. estimates that children eat as much as a quarter pound of coal-tar based dyes each year.[55] The annual consumption of yellow numbers five and six, and red number three in 1984 was 3.4 million pounds. Yellow number five and six have already been banned in Norway, due to known carcinogenicity.[56]

Red dye numbers three, eight, nine, 19, 33, 36, 37; blue number one and two; orange number 17; yellow number five and six; green number three—the color assortment of coal-tar based dyes listed under the Food, Drug and Cosmetic Act could rival the selection at your favorite home decorating center. The above dyes have been targeted by "Public Citizen," a consumer group based in Washington D.C., in an effort to have them banned from further use in the marketplace for reasons of health, either as potential carcinogens or as allergens.

Currently, red dyes number 17, 19 and 37, and orange number 17 are permitted for external use only in cosmetics and toiletries. Red dye numbers eight and nine are permitted in lipsticks and red dye number three in foods.[57]

Around 1960, suspicions rose about the possible carcinogenity of red dye number two. Laboratory tests conducted in the Soviet Union and published in 1971 showed that this dye could induce birth defects and cause cancer. Red dye number two was finally banned in 1976 when extensive tests on laboratory rats showed that it is metabolized by every organ in the body, that it can cause genetic mutations, and that it causes multiple tumors in rats over a two year period. Between 1960 and 1976, however, the Food and Drug Administration gave 15 extensions of this product's provisional status before it was banned.

Red dye number two has been superseded by red dye number 40; its use is now so widespread in the United States that it has become the standard coloring agent in a multitude of foods, such as imitation fruit drinks, candy, ice cream, hot dogs, and even pet foods. However, there are eight countries that have not approved the use of this dye: Canada, Sweden, Norway, Japan, Italy, Israel, France, Austria, Great Britain, Australia. Their reasons: "Only limited information is available on this substance."

Incidental Additives

Methylene chloride, one of the solvents mentioned in this chapter as a chemical, is used to extract caffeine from coffee. However, many coffee makers are now using less methylene chloride—a suspected carcinogen—for decaffeinated coffee.

Daminozide is used on the farm for uniform ripening of apples and other crops. Some people are calling these "embalmed" apples. Studies have shown an increased risk of cancer in animals tested with daminozide.

Food Preservatives. BHA, BHT are two compounds used as preservatives (antioxidants) in breakfast cereals, vegetable oils, processed meats, snacks and spices to prolong shelf life and in prevention of rancidity. There is evidence of the BHA and BHT compounds causing cancer in test animals according to the World Health Organization's agency for Research on Cancer.

For information on organic foods, contact Joseph Rogers, D.O., at Safe Foods, Inc., 12499 Delta Drive, Taylor, MI 48180, (313) 946-6446.

DIETARY HABITS AND CANCER

Cancer development may be triggered by the following:

- A diet that is too high in calories.
- A sedentary life style.
- Overconsumption of certain foods, especially containing saturated fats and cholesterol in animal fats.
- The presence of alcohol, coffee, food additives.
- Substances that may contaminate food by mold, curing or fermentation.
- Foods cooked in certain ways: smoked, charbroiled, barbecued, etc.
- Carcinogens formed by the body's own natural processes.
- The use of alcohol, especially in conjunction with smoking.
- Beverages that have been artificially sweetened and dyed, especially if consumed in childhood, or during pregnancy.

The average American can exercise some control over this disease by making a few important and informed choices in the supermarket and at mealtime.

Fats and Calories

To make sure that every meal and snack contain no more than 20 percent calories from fat: read the product label, which should list the grams of fat per serving, multiply by nine (the number of calories in each gram of fat), and divide by the number of calories per serving.

For example, there are five grams of fat per serving of low fat two percent milk, and 120 calories in a one cup serving:

5 (grams fat) x 9 (calories/gram) = 45 calories from fat;
45 divided by 120 = 37.5 percent calories from fat.

Hard cheeses, with about 73 percent calories from fat, are particularly ruinous to fat-calorie-cholesterol watchers. Cheeses that are labelled "low-fat" cottage cheese or "part-skim" mozzarella, feta, or ricotta and neufchatyl cream cheese are lower in fat content. Restrict the use of other cheeses such as parmesan to a "sprinkling". Read labels, and watch the sodium content of these products.

Fiber

The average American falls short of the National Cancer Institute's recommendations of at least 25-35 grams of fiber each day, and ideally 50 to 60 grams. You do not need to consume unprocessed bran or other unpalatable foods. Many ethnic foods have a high-fiber content naturally: polenta, bulgur wheat, corn and whole wheat tortillas, and whole wheat pasta.

Note the difference between whole wheat products and cracked wheat or wheat products which are usually made with enriched white wheat flour and contain virtually no fiber per serving.

Vegetables

Soups and salads, made with fresh vegetables and fruits, are excellent ways to increase intake of vitamins A and C, reduce fat and also increase fiber.

Stocks and broths—the basis of any good soup—should be cooked at a low simmer, otherwise the vegetables turn to mush and are unpalatable. To remove fat, strain through a mesh strainer and two layers of cheese cloth. Chill the soup and skim off any remaining fat that has hardened on the top.

A rule of thumb for salads: the darker and more colorful the lettuce leaf, the more vitamins it contains.

The oil in salad dressings is 100 percent fat. A painless way to cut the amount of salad oil is to use chicken or vegetable broth as a "filler." Using broth or non-fat yogurt as a substitute for oil is easier on the taste buds than bottled low-cal dressing.

For cooked vegetables—less is more; less water and less cooking time leave more nutrients. Stir-frying and steaming are the best methods for retaining nutrients.

Do not overlook the lowly potato. The literal translation for potato in French is "the earth's apple"—an apt name for a vegetable so rich in vitamin A, C, and fiber. It can be used as a thickening agent in soups and stews along with many other modes of preparation.

Because vitamin C is so perishable, there is more of it in the juice of a freshly sliced orange than from a glass of reconstituted orange juice.

Protein and Fats

The average American eats more meat than is necessary for a balanced diet and probably takes too large a serving. No matter what size portion you serve yourself at dinnertime, it can probably stand trimming. One serving consisting of three ounces of red meat, or four ounces of chicken or fish. This amount supplies an adult female with 62 percent of her daily protein requirement, and an adult male with 49 percent.

MEATS TO EAT OFTEN: white meat of turkey or chicken without skin, white fish (some examples are halibut, sole, flounder, perch, shark, swordfish), water-packed tuna or salmon, shellfish such as clams and mussels, lobster, veal, and scallopine of beef or veal.

MEATS TO EAT SOMETIMES: lean sirloin of beef, ground round, dark meat of poultry, pink or red salmon, flank steak, lean cuts of veal and lamb.

SPECIAL OCCASIONS: standing rib roasts, lean pork, shrimp, veal roasts, lamb chops.

Nutrition from each of the four food groups is necessary for vitality and health. The objective is to rearrange the balance, favoring vitamin, nutrient and fiber rich foods over foods high in fat and cholesterol or enhanced with chemicals.

Healthy Menus

The following are examples of daily meal plans, one designed for adults and one for children. These can be used as examples for you and your family of a balanced daily diet which combines optimum nutritional values with simplicity.

HEALTHY MENUS
by Mary Hillcoat, R.D.

ADULT MENU

BREAKFAST Orange juice, ½ cup
Egg Substitute, ½ cup
Mixed Grain Toast, 2 slices
Skim Milk, 1 cup
Tea

LUNCH Tuna Pita Sandwich, 1
Fresh Pineapple with Skim Milk Yogurt, 1 cup
Skim Milk, 1 cup
Tea

DINNER Chicken Stir Fry on Wild Rice, 1 serving
Waldorf Salad, 1 Cup
Angel Food Cake with Blueberry topping, 1 serving
Skim Milk, 1 cup
Tea

SNACK Air-popped popcorn with Onion powder, 2 cups

ANALYSIS

Calories	2,425
Fat	60.4 G
Dietary Fiber	32.1 G
Cholesterol	101 Mg.
Vitamin A	1,913 RE
Vitamin C	522 Mg.
Vitamin E	28.3 Mg.
Calcium	1,610 Mg.
Selenium	118 Mcg.
Calories from Fats	20 Percent

CHILDREN'S MENU

BREAKFAST   Fresh Orange, 1
                 Egg Substitute, ¼ cup
                 Mixed Grain Toast, 1 slice
                 Strawberry Jam, 1 tsp
                 Skim Milk, 1 cup

LUNCH   Peanut butter and Marmalade on Mixed
                 Grain Bread Sandwich, 1
                 Carrot Sticks, 1 carrot
                 Bartlett Pear, 1
                 Skim Milk, 1 cup

SNACK   Raisin Toast, 1 slice
                 Skim Milk, 1 cup

DINNER   Chicken Stir Fry on Wild Rice, ½ serving
                 Waldorf Salad, ½ cup
                 Angel Food Cake with Blueberry Topping, 1 serving
                 Skim Milk, 1 cup

SNACK   Air-popped Popcorn with Onion powder, 2 cups
                 Skim Milk, 1 cup

ANALYSIS

Calories	2,185
Fat	67 G
Dietary Fiber	33.2 G
Cholesterol	79.4 Mg
Vitamin A	3,485 RE
Vitamin C	130 Mg
Vitamin E	20.9 Mg
Calcium	1,900 Mg
Selenium	106 Mcg
Calories from Fats	27 Percent

CANCER INHIBITORS

The idea that we can eat to prevent cancer sounds exciting, but at the moment, it is not a realistic possibility. Some chemical agents have been found to inhibit the action of carcinogens in animals. Much research in this area has been done by Dr. L. W. Wattenberg. Presently the National Cancer Institute is conducting long-term trials with some of these compounds.

Natural cancer inhibitors come in four categories, as illustrated by the following table.

NATURAL CANCER INHIBITORS[58]

Category	Foods	Inhibit

I. ISOTHIOCYANATES	Cauliflower
	Broccoli
	Cabbage
	Brussels Sprouts
		Nitrosamines
		Aflatoxin
		Benzopyrene,
		  tar compounds
		  found in smoke

II. ANTIOXIDANTS	Vitamins A,C,E	Anti-cancerous powers
Sulphydryl Compounds, Selenium & Curcumin	Garlic & Onions	Have anti-cancerous properties
Curcumin	Tumeric	Has anti-cancerous properties
Substance P	Hot Peppers	Blocks Benzopyrene

III. WASHING
    AND COOKING
	Cooking
	Mushrooms
		Destroys
		  many toxins

IV. FIBER	Grains Vegetables Fruits	Reduces risk of Colon Cancer

CHAPTER SIX NOTES

1. Peter Greenwald, "Manipulation of Nutrients to Prevent Cancer," *Hospital Practice*, (May 1984)
2. Saul Gusberg, "The Individual at High Risk for Endometrial Carcinoma," *American Journal of Obstetrics and Gynecology*, (Nov. 1976)
3. Philip Cole, and Daniel Cramer, "Diet and Cancer of the Endocrine Target Organs," *Cancer*, (July 1977)

4. *Journal of the American Medical Association,* (July 28, 1989)

5. Kathleen Tyndall, "Obesity isn't a State but a Killing Disease, NIH Panel Says," *Family Practice News,* (April 1, 1985)

6. Ralph Paffenbarger, et.al. *New England Journal of Medicine,* (March 1986)

7. Rose Frisch, *Physician Washington Report,* (March 6, 1986)

8. Steven Blair, et.al. *Journal of the American Medical Association,* (Nov. 3, 1989)

9. Slattery, Martha; Ana W. Sorenson, and Marilyn H. Ford, "Dietary Calcium Intake as Mitigating Factor in Colon Cancer," *American Journal of Epidemiology,* Vol. 128, (1988)

10. Snowden, David A.; Rolland C. Phillips and Warren Choi, "Diet, Obesity and Risk of Fatal Prostate Cancers," *American Journal of Epidemiology,* Vol. 120, #2, 1984

11. Ryan, *Journal of the American Medical Association,* (July 19, 1985)

12. Michael Bunk, and Richard Rivlin, "Nutrition and Prevention of Cancer: Some Comments on Recent Developments," *Current Concepts and Perspectives on Nutrition,* Vol. 6, #1. (March 1, 1987)

13. *Journal of the American Medical Association,* (Jan. 17, 1986)

14. Dennis Burkitt, "The Bran Hypothesis," *Harvard Medical School Health Letter,* (Sept. 1980)

15. *Ibid.*

16. Johnson, *Medical Tribune,* (June 10, 1987)

17. Erik Bjelke, "Dietary Vitamin A and Lung Cancer," *International Journal of Cancer,* 15:561-565, (1975)

18. Ward Hinds, *American Journal of Epidemiology.* Vol. 119, #2

19. Dorothy Mackerras, *American Journal of Epidemiology,* 128:5, (1988)

20. Paul Stehr, *American Journal of Epidemiology,* 121:1, (1985)

21. Gerald Shklar, *New England Journal of Medicine,* (Dec. 11, 1986)

22. R. E. Clark, *Lancet,* (April 4, 1987)

23. *Medical Tribune,* (March 17, 1985)

24. S. Wassertheil-Smoller, *American Journal of Epidemiology,* Vol. 114, (1981)

25. Robert E. Wittes, *New England Journal of Medicine,* (Jan.17, 1985)

26. Saxon Graham, "A Dietary Prevention of Cancer," *Epidemiological Reviews,* Vol. 5, (1983)

27. *American Journal of Epidemiology,* (1981)

28. Garry Duthie, *Prevention Magazine,* (March 1989)

29. Paul Knekt, et. al., *American Journal of Epidemiology,* (1988)

30. Duthie, *Prevention Magazine,* (March 1989)

31. Slattery, et.al., *American Journal of Epidemiology,* Vol. 128, #3, (1988)

32. Vernon Young, "Selenium: A Case for Its Essentiality in Men," *New England Journal of Medicine,* (May 14, 1981)

33. *Journal of the American Medical Association,* (Dec. 26, 1986)

34. Board of Trustees of the American Medical Association. *Journal of the American Medical Association,* (Sept. 19, 1986)

35. James Chow, *Diagnosis*, (Oct. 1984)

36. *Medical Tribune*, (Jan. 21, 1983)

37. Hartge, P. et al., *Journal of the National Cancer Institute*, 70, (June 1983)

38. D.B. Thomas; Charles N. Uhl; P. Hartge, "Bladder Cancer and Alcoholic Beverage Consumption," *American Journal of Epidemiology*, Vol. 118 #5 (1983)

39. James Breeden, "Alcohol-Alcoholism and Cancer," *Medical Clinics of North America*, Vol. 68 #1, (Jan, 1984)

40. Robert A. Hiatt, and Richard D. Bawol, *American Journal of Epidemiology*, 120 (1984)

41. Walter C. Willett, et.al. *New England Journal of Medicine*, (May 7, 1987)

42. *Journal of the American Medical Association*, (Sept 19, 1986)

43. Brian McMahon, et al., "Coffee and Cancer of Pancreas," *New England Journal of Medicine*, (March 1981)

44. Lorraine Marrett, et.al. "Coffee Drinking and Bladder Cancer in Connecticut," *American Journal of Epidemiology*, Vol. 117, #2. (Feb. 1983)

45. J.P. Minton, et.al., *Cancer Journal*, (April 1, 1989)

46. P.N. McGee, and J.M. Barnes, *British Journal of Cancer*, (1956)

47. *Medical Tribune Report* (Jan. 7, 1987)

48. R.O. Sinnhuber, et.al., *Journal of the National Cancer Institute*, Vol. 41, (Sept. 1968)

49. *Medical Tribune*, (January, 1989)

50. *Medical World News*, (August 16, 1982)

51. *American Medical News*, (Jan. 11, 1985)

52. Council on Scientific Affairs Report, *Journal of the American Medical Association*, (Nov. 8, 1985)

53. W. Allman, "Pesticides - An Unhealthy Dependence?" *Science*, (Oct. 1985)

54. Council on Scientific Affairs, *Journal of American Medical Association*, (July 19, 1985)

55. Epstein, *The Politics of Cancer*. p.181

56. *American Medical News*, (Jan. 11, 1985)

57. *Physician's Washington Report*, (Nov. 1984)

58. Devra Lee Davis, National Academy of the Sciences, *Environmental Health Digest*, (Feb. 1990)

CHAPTER SEVEN

HORMONES AND DRUGS

In the year 1916, researchers named Lathrop and Loeb demonstrated that the castration of mice prevented breast cancer.[1] This study was the first clue that breast cancer was hormone dependent; we now know that at least one-third of breast cancers are hormone dependent.

In 1932, other researchers, such as Dr. Lecassagne, demonstrated that estrogen injections caused breast cancer in mice. Dr. Huggins reported improvement in prostate cancer patients with estrogens in 1940. After the war, biotechnology improved, and the relationship of hormones to cancer became more clear. Synthetic hormones were developed shortly thereafter.

According to Dr. John Berg of the University of Iowa, it is now estimated that up to 36 percent of female cancers and 27 percent of male cancers, excluding skin cancer, are hormone dependent.[2] A person's own hormones seem to control cancer formation as well as synthetic hormones that are introduced into the body. Hormones appear to set the stage for formation of cancer, which makes them cancer promoters in general. They can also cause cancer in the offspring of mothers who are exposed to them during pregnancy, as in the case of the synthetic estrogen hormone DES.

FINE TUNING A HUMAN SYMPHONY

Like a finely tuned orchestra, the balance of hormones in the human body is exquisitely sensitive. To understand how unbalanced hormones can set the stage for cancer, it is important to understand something of how they work. The word "hormone" is derived from the Greek word for messenger. Unlike the nervous system, hormones are not connected through tissues; instead, they relay their messages via the bloodstream from the body's 13 endocrine glands: the pancreas, the pineal, the pituitary, the thyroid, the thymus, two adrenals, four parathyroids, and two sex gonads (ovaries in females, testes in males).

Hormonal activities are regulated by the pituitary, or the master gland, which acts on messages received from the small whitish area of the brain called the hypothalamus. The hypothalamus, the seat of emotions and thought processes, is the real conductor of this human symphony.

The flow of hormones stimulates many organs, tissues and functions in the human body. Most important for our discussion on cancer are the female hormone estrogen and the male hormone androgen, which regulate all aspects of human sexual and reproductive functions. Supplies of these hormones change during adolescence and at menopause.

The body's own supply of hormones can now be replaced, enhanced, adjusted, or regulated from the outside, either with natural or synthetic hormones. As with any medication, the physician must make a judgement of the benefits versus the risk of prescribing hormones. In our consumer oriented society, physicians should warn patients that they may pay a high price for feeling good, feeling young and feeling strong through medication. While hormones do not cause cancer, they may set the stage for the promotion of cancer.

OVEREATING AND OVERHEATING

Geographical patterns of hormone dependent cancers worldwide suggests that they are cancers of affluence. As people become more affluent, they eat more animal meat and fats. It is apparent that as the fat in the diet increases, the evidence of hormone-dependent cancers like breast, uterus, ovaries, prostate and testes, increase. For example, moving from Japan through Asia to Western Europe and North America the incidence of these cancers continues to increase. Breast cancer is ten times more common in the United States than in Japan. By the same token, as the Japanese move to the United States, their hormone dependent cancer rates go up. These geographic cancer patterns for hormone dependent cancers are closely related to the patterns of bowel cancer—which has also been shown to be related to diets high in animal fat and cholesterol.

It appears that high levels of animal fat in the diet results in an over-function of the hormonal system and over-growth of the hormone dependant areas in the body, such as breasts, ovaries and uterus in women and prostate and testicles in men. A high fat diet results in increased blood level of estrogen in females, while a vegetarian diet lowers hormone levels.[3] The rates of breast cancer in vegetarian American women such as Seventh Day Adventists are only 60-80 percent of the rates of the general American population.

Obese women have high levels of estrogen because their body fat acts as a conversion factory—converting the androgens (male hormones) produced by the ovaries and adrenal glands into the cancer promoting hormone estrone. Accordingly, obese, hypertensive and diabetic women have a high incidence of cancer of the uterus. A study by Dr. Flora Lubin of Tel Aviv University,[4] showed that 50 percent of the older women in western countries are 20 percent or more overweight. If this excessive weight were reduced, deaths from breast cancer would be reduced by at least 30 percent.

SYNTHETIC HORMONES

Over 100 million prescriptions for hormones have been written by American physicians since 1970. Chances are that if you are a middle-aged American woman (aged 45-60) facing discomfort from menopause, a young woman in the peak years of fertility, or a pregnant woman threatening to abort, you have received one of these prescriptions. The results have been dramatic. Although hormones are effective, they are suspected in some cases to be cancer promoters.

The quick results of hormones do not affect women alone. Young American males, ranging from high-school football players or international Olympians to worshippers of Sylvester Stallone and Arnold Schwartzenegger—anyone obsessed with obtaining a more muscular physique or a better athletic performance—have been taking anabolic steroids (called DECAS) at an alarming rate. These hormones work: within two weeks, a body-builder can see his muscles ripple and bulge, though a good deal of the results are from water retention. Since these hormones are not manufactured for body building, those who use them for aesthetic purposes usually have to guess at the correct dosages.

Americans of all ages ingest hormones daily through the synthetic food additives which are used to fatten the cattle, poultry and other livestock in our diets. It has been estimated that a beef animal given the synthetic estrogen DES as an additive to its diet reaches a market weight of 1,000 pounds about 35 days sooner than an untreated animal, saving nearly 500 pounds of feed per animal. Direct savings to the feedlot industry because of DES use were estimated at over 90 million dollars per year in 1974.

Even the family cat or dog is not spared. Packaged pet foods, usually made from the discarded by-products of meat and poultry, contain excessively high amounts of residual hormones.

FEMALE HORMONES

Contemporary American culture places a high value on feeling vital, alive, youthful, vigorous and competitive. The media and the marketplace have ennobled this ideal of human physical perfection, and have made it a consumer product. Writer Blair Sabol has described contemporary Americans as the "gym generation" in her book *The Body of America.*[5]

Next to tranquilizers, female sex hormones are the second most frequently prescribed drugs in America today. Their use is widespread, and most Americans take them with a sense of security, believing that they have been tested, researched, and documented. Prescriptions are usually given for healthy people to make them feel and look even healthier.

Yet, as early as 1896, researchers suspected that there was a link between hormonal activity and cancer growth. When women with advanced breast cancer had their ovaries removed, they experienced a temporary regression of the disease. In men, too, castration (by cutting off the supply of the male hormone testosterone) has been a well-known means of treating prostate cancer.

By the 1930s, animal researchers knew that hormone therapy could prevent ovulation in rabbits. There were rumored to be crude experiments in hormonal birth control in the concentration camps of Nazi Germany. By the mid 1940s, the first synthetic estrogen had been developed and was called DES. It was marketed by dozens of drug companies for preventing threatened abortions.

There are millions of Americans who wish to deny the connection between hormones and cancer. It must be understood that hormones, when used as steroids, as oral contraceptives, or for estrogen replacement therapy, can play havoc with a very delicate and sensitive harmony in human biological functions.

The Birth Control Pill

In the United States since 1960, over 30 different formulations of oral contraceptives have appeared on the market. About 12 million women in the United States (half single and half married) use them

145

regularly.[6] Though the statistical population fluctuates because many women do not take oral contraceptives all of their child-bearing years, these women represent a consumer market in excess of 100 million dollars each year.[7] Over 63 million married women use the pill worldwide, according to a Popular Information Program at Johns Hopkins School of Public Health.

There has been an ongoing debate about the role of birth control pills in causation of breast cancer since they were first introduced in the early 1960s. Breast cancer is a common disease in Western women, affecting one in ten, and there is mounting evidence, as described earlier, that hormones do have a role in its causation.[8] A recent Cancer and Steroid Hormone Study has provided reassurance to women who used birth control pills for up to 15 years that they are not at high risk for breast cancer.[9]

A study conducted in the 1970s by Centers for Disease Control and National Institute of Child Health and Human Development analyzed the use of oral contraceptives on the incidence of breast cancer. It was determined that there was no increased risk of breast cancer connected with pill use, but the study stated that its data did not go beyond 15 years of follow up.[10]

Particularly regarding cancer, the benefits of the pill seem to outweigh the risks, especially when one considers the changes oral contraceptives have undergone in their lifetime. Thirty different oral contraceptive products have been introduced since the pill's inception, evolving from the "sequential" type to the current "combination" type. The amount of estrogen in today's oral contraceptives is actually ten times lower than in the early pills of the 1960s.

The old, sequential type of birth control pills, were found to increase the risk of uterine cancer in the mid-seventies. They were discontinued in 1976 and were withdrawn from the market in United States and Canada. In these pills, the three phase cycle consisted of 1) estrogens for two weeks, 2) estrogen plus progesterone for one week, 3) nothing for one week, and then the cycle was repeated.

Dr. Barbara Hulka of the University of North Carolina believes that the present type of birth control pill, in which estrogen and progesterone are combined, reduces the risk of cancer of the uterus.[11] The combination type of birth control pills has also been found to protect against cancer of the ovaries, according to the recent Cancer and Steroid Hormone Study.[12] They reduce the risk of ovarian cancer by 40 percent in women 20-54 years of age, even if they are used for only a few months. The researchers estimated that birth control pills prevented 1,700 cases of ovarian cancer in 1982 alone—a remarkable statistic. Thus, a pill relying on the combination of estrogen and progestin has been found to be much safer, both for the prevention of pregnancy and the prevention of cancer, than a pill that juggles these two hormones sequentially.

Nevertheless, the statistical studies linking oral contraceptives to heart disease, hypertension, diabetes, and to cancer have been playing "catch up"—in other words, follow-up studies may not have had a long enough time to tell the whole story. Studies also have to consider the long term effects of both the sequential type and the combination type oral contraceptive. The most damaging evidence against use of "the pill" can be found in several recently completed studies. One, conducted by the United States Center for Disease Control in Atlanta, was on 5,600 women who had used oral contraceptives for 12 years; they were found to have 12 times the risk of breast cancer compared to women who had not used them. In another, an English team found that women in their 30s had three times the risk of breast cancer as compared to control groups of women who did not use the pill.

Female hormones do not cause melanoma, but they do play an adverse role in melanoma patients. Patients with melanoma or with a history of melanoma should not take birth control pills or other female hormone preparations or steroids. The risk of developing cancer increases with longer use: two-and-a-half times for use of five to nine years, and three-and-a-half times for use of ten years or longer, according to Dr. Elizabeth Holly at the University of California.[13] Evidence is accumulating that birth control pills also have a role in promoting liver cancer and benign tumors. It is prudent for patients on birth control pills to have liver function tests for early detection of liver tumors.[14]

There have been many studies done in the United States and in other countries on the subject of oral contraceptives; the conflicting results of these studies indicate the need for continued research.

Estrogen Replacement Therapy (ERT)—The 'Forever Feminine' Pill

Estrogens were first put on the market for post-menopausal syndrome in 1942 in the United States. In keeping with the "youth culture" of the 1960s, it was common practice to use ERT. Use continued into the 70s. Because 40 million women in the United States are aged 50 or over, the market for estrogen replacement therapy is huge.[15]

Between 1964 and 1975, the prescriptions for ERT increased from nine million to 25 million, while the number of users increased from 1.7 to five million. But a 1981 survey showed that after 1975, because of published reports linking estrogen levels with cancer of the uterus, ERT prescriptions decreased to 12 million.[16]

The estrogens are commonly used for well-known post-menopausal symptom. "Flushes and flashes" are no joke to the women who go through them. Approximately 75 percent of post-menopausal women experience them, but only 15-20 percent look for treatment. Estrogens are also used in the treatment of osteoporosis and for health of the genitalia and bladder.

Many physicians have reported how gratifying it was to treat symptomatic menopausal women with estrogen. They see immediate reduction in the assorted complaints of hot flashes, depression, itching, vaginal atrophy, insomnia, and osteoporosis.

Estrogen replacement therapy (ERT) has little use in preventing wrinkles, forestalling aging, or making anyone more fit for the gym. Unfortunately, it is occasionally used for these results anyway. By 1975, the *New England Journal of Medicine* had documented that endometrial cancer increased five to 14 times among ERT users as compared to non-users. The dosage and duration of use were major factors in promoting cancer, and some women had been on ERT for as long as ten years.

Since cancer of the uterus and breast both create estrogen dependent tumors, concerns about breast cancer rose with use of post-menopausal estrogens. Dr. Louise Brinton and associates of the National Cancer Institute found a higher risk of breast cancer in all users of menopausal estrogens in a 1981 study. According to the study, the risk increased two or three fold in women who had used estrogen for ten or more years, who had ovaries removed, or who had a family history of breast cancer. The risk multiplied four times in longer term users.[17]

Estrogen is now combined with progesterone to make "mini pills" which do not seem to increase the risk of cancer.[18] If you are taking the "mini pill," you should have an annual breast and pelvic exam, a Pap smear and a mini-D and C.

If estrogens are used alone, they should be used in small doses for short periods of time, and under medical supervision. They should not be used in any form if the patient has a medical history of breast cancer, uterine cancer, heart attack, stroke or any undiagnosed vaginal bleeding.

DES: "The Bitter Pill"

DES is the grandmother of all synthetic estrogen hormones and was developed in the late 1930s. Robert Meyers describes the DES story in remarkable detail in his book, *DES — The Bitter Pill*.[19] He writes that a Boston obstetrician named George Van Siclen Smith started experimenting with the drug when he noticed hormone levels in pregnant women dropped dramatically when they were threatening to miscarry. He called it initially the "Smith & Smith Regimen," named after himself and his wife and co-worker in 1948. Later many other physicians used it on their patients to prevent miscarriages. DES became widely used in the United States and to a lesser extent in Australia and England. The use of DES continued until the mid-1950s, when Drs. W.J. Dieckman and associates found DES use to be of no value in pregnancy.[20] After this report the use of DES for women declined markedly, but its other uses, such as an additive for cattle feed, continued.

In 1966, a 15-year old girl turned up at Massachusetts General Hospital with a diagnosis of adenocarcinoma of the vagina, a cancer that is found in glandular tissue. Normal vaginas have no glandular tissue, but this young girl had many tiny glands in her vagina. No one under the age of 25 had ever been diagnosed with this disease at Massachusetts General. A "mini-epidemic" of cancer of the vagina was found in many young women whose mothers had taken DES.

In 1971, a report was published in the *New England Journal of Medicine* by Dr. Arthur Herbst, establishing that hormones not only helped cancer grow, but could also cause cancer in a newly forming fetus. The most sinister aspect of DES was the delayed effect; the drug could cause cancer in cervix and vagina a decade or more after contact.

Given to nearly two million women in the United States, DES was removed from the marketplace by the FDA in 1971. But its memories—bitter memories—linger on. There have been lawsuits in every state, but treatment, not blame, is what matters most to the innocent victims.

With funding from the National Cancer Institute and the American Cancer Society, Dr. Herbst has established a DES Information Center, listing all women born after 1940 who have had DES-related cancer. There are 500 names on this list. So far, a quarter of these women, daughters of the DES recipients, have had reoccurrences or have died.

It is estimated that between 100,000 to 500,000 DES-exposed women were born in 1960-70. Of the daughters who have had follow-up exams thus far, almost 100 percent show vaginal and cervical abnormalities if their mothers took DES before the eighth week of pregnancy. DES usually affects women between seven and 31 years, with a peak age of 19 years.

Dr. Stanley Robboy and his associates reviewed the incidence of cancer to be one to five percent in patients with dysplasia (abnormal lining) on the Pap smear of a woman exposed to DES.[21] According to Dr. Sandra Melnick, the incidence of cancer due to DES exposure in a woman in her mid-30s is one in 1,000, which makes this cancer rare.

DES sons also exhibit reproductive abnormalities such as undersized testes or penises, testicular mass or cysts, along with undescended testicles and testicular cancer.[22] Few have conceived children, so it is

149

unclear whether any DES males have been rendered sterile. Only time will tell.

Recommended Treatment for DES Exposure

For daughters exposed to DES during pregnancy, yearly check ups should start at age 14. More information about DES can be obtained by contacting:

> DES, Office of Cancer Communication
> National Cancer Institute, Building 31
> Bethesda, MD 20892
>   Telephone: 1 (800) 4-CANCER

Or Reading:

> *DES, The Bitter Pill*, by Robert Meyers.
> Seaview/Putnam, New York, 1983.

STEROIDS: TALES FROM THE LOCKER ROOM

In the United States, interest in physical fitness has intensified since 1970. First it was jogging, then in the 80s body building became popular. Along with the gyms and health clubs came the desire for a "quick fix," the genie in the bottle, magic pills to enhance the body.

Steroids are derivatives of male hormones. Male hormone was first used by Russian athletes during the 1956 Olympics. Derivatives of male hormone were used primarily by physicians to build up the emaciated bodies of cancer patients. Later they were picked up for use by professional athletes and football players.

Steroids used to create an instant powerful-looking body became available both in pill and injection form. They are used in regimens called "stacking" or "pyramids" or "stacking the pyramids." Stacking combines two agents; pyramids gradually increases doses; and stacking the pyramids combines multiple agents in increasing fashion. According to one young regular at the gym, within a couple of weeks steroids can make arm muscles bulge out of shirt sleeves. Much of this is water that is held in the tissues, and traces of the drug can linger for up to a year after its use.

The sport of body-building entered a new realm of popularity and respectability about ten years ago when Sylvester Stallone talked candidly about his preparations for the movie role of "Rocky." Many of Stallone's clones talk about their admiration for their hero, or the yearly competition for the title of Mr. Olympia and the 55,000 dollar first prize that goes with it. They do not talk about steroids that they may or may not be using.

Of the 35 million Americans who pump iron, medical experts Kenneth Kashkin and Herbert Kleber believe that about one million use illegal steroids, either by mouth or injection, and spend about 100 million dollars on the black market.[23] Out of these users, 250,000 are high school seniors. A recent study found that almost seven percent of high school seniors had used anabolic steroids, coming to an estimated one-half million high school males who are using or have used anabolic steroids.[24] Some individuals are spending as much as 20,000 dollars a year on them, taking doses between 750 mg. and 3700 mg. a week. It takes the normal functions of the human body a year to produce that amount, at an average rate of about four milligrams daily.

A scandal ensued at the 1988 Summer Olympic Games when Canadian sprinter Ben Johnson lost his gold medal after testing positive for steroids. Athletes in other sports, such as football, have also been caught using steroids. With the new awareness of steroids, testing has become more rigorous.

The complications brought on by steroid over-use are many. High blood pressure, blood clots, decreased testicular size, sterility, diabetes, pre-cancerous liver tumors called adenomas, which are sharply on the increase, kidney disease, and liver cancers have been reported. A body builder in England reportedly died of liver cancer after using steroids. According to the report by Drs. Kashkin and Kleber, steroids appear to be addicting because of their psychological effects.

MEDICATIONS AND SECOND TUMORS

There are many medications other than hormones which can promote the development of cancer. A number of agents fall into this category: chemotherapeutic agents, immunosuppressive drugs, miscellaneous drugs such as Phenacetin used in headache remedies, and chloramphenicol, an antibiotic.

Chemotherapy

One of the minor causes of cancer are the agents in chemotherapy, responsible for one percent of total cancer occurrences in the United States, according to estimates by Drs. T. Thomas Taylor and Adelbert E. Wade, of the College of Pharmacy at the University of Georgia.[25] Chemotherapy was discovered during World War II when it was noted that soldiers exposed to mustard gas had low white blood cell counts. The idea of using nitrogen mustard emerged as an experimental treatment for leukemia and is still used for the disease.

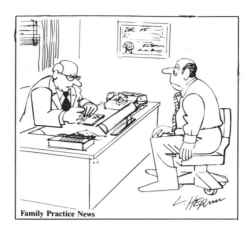

"The trouble is in your side, so
I'm giving you something
that has side effects!"

Reprinted from Family Practice News, March 15-31, 1985, ©1985,
Fairchild Publications, a division of Capital Cities Media, Inc., and by
permission of Mr. Leonard Herman.

In the last 20 years there has been a marked improvement in the treatment of cancer patients with chemotherapy and radiation. Many patients are living today due to a cure or palliation of their cancer. However, chemotherapy does not come without a serious price. One of the more serious effects is an increased risk of cancer from the treatment itself, although many times it is nearly impossible to tell if a cancer was actually caused by treatment.

One critical factor in chemotherapy is the age of the patient. The young seem to be especially vulnerable in terms of damage from chemotherapy, and are at high risk for breast, lung, stomach cancers and sarcomas, say researchers Diane Young and George P. Canellos in *Medical Clinics of North America*.[26] The number of such patients with a second cancer is also going to be high; Drs. Anna T. Meadows and Jeffery Silber of the Children's Hospital of Philadelphia estimate that by 1990, one in every 1,000 young adults by age 20 will be a survivor of a childhood cancer.[27] Not only are these young adults at high risk for second cancers, but their children also have a high risk for developing a childhood cancer.

The examples listed below are of secondary cancers caused by treatment of the initial cancer as cited in the article by Drs. Young and Canellos.

1. *Acute Leukemia (Non Lymphatic Type) as a secondary cancer occurs after:*

   —Treatment of Hodgkin's disease and acute leukemia with chemotherapy and radiation in five to ten percent of cases over a period of ten years. In younger patients the risk of secondary cancer can be increased by 30-40 percent.

   —Non-Hodgkin Lymphoma with chemotherapy and radiation treatment.

   —Multiple myeloma with chemotherapy and radiation.

   —Ovarian cancer treated with chemotherapy.

   —Breast, gastrointestinal and testicular cancer treatment with chemotherapy.

2. *Non-Hodgkin Lymphoma is sometimes seen after treatment of Hodgkin's Disease.*

3. *Solid tumors found in the body treated by chemotherapy.*

The risk of secondary cancer in children appears to be 12 percent in children treated before 1971, and eight percent from more recent statistics. Over all, these figures amount to a 10-20 times greater risk than for the general population.[28] Efforts are being made to reduce this risk by using new drug combinations.

Not only are patients at high risk for getting these secondary cancers, but the manufacturers of these anti-cancer drugs, the pharmacists who prepare the solutions and nurses who administer them, all increase their risk through exposure. Recent studies have shown a high rate of miscarriage among chemotherapy nurses and breakdown residuals of these chemotherapy products have been noted in their urine.

Chemotherapy should be seen as a double-edged sword, able to cure, but also able to cause cancer.

Immunosuppressive Drugs

Patients who receive organ transplants are often given immunosuppressive drugs to prevent rejection of the organ. There is a danger that the body may view the new organ as a foreign substance and try to get rid of it. Cyclosporine, used for kidney, heart and liver transplants, is an immunosuppressive drug often given to patients for this reason. However, cyclosporine has been linked with lymphatic cancer called lymphoma. Physicians can reduce the risk for lymphoma by having a "well-matched donor organ and the lowest possible effective immuno-suppressant doses." Heart transplant patients who were treated with cyclosporine seem to run the highest risk for acquiring lymphoma.[29]

An immunosuppressive drug such as penicillamine therapy has been used for treating Wilson's disease (a metabolic defect in copper metabolism) and for other diseases. This drug may also be associated with the development of leukemia.[30]

PUVA

In 1974, Dr. Parrish at the University of Michigan in Ann Arbor, started a treatment for psoriasis, a skin condition, which included applications of PUVA, a tar compound, with "light treatments" or ultraviolet light from sunlamps. These patients were found to be at almost three times the risk for skin cancer by a multicenter study headed by Dr. Robert Stern and associates of the Harvard Medical School.[31]

Phenacetin and Pain Medications

People who use pain medications frequently, either with or without phenacetin, have two times the risk of renal pelvic cancer; their risk increases to somewhere between six and 16 times with heavy use of pain medication. More recent studies have found that women between 20-49 with bladder cancer were 6.5 times as likely to say they had used analgesics with phenacetin than age-matched controls.[32]

The medications mentioned below are suspected to have possible links with cancer:[33]

Phenylbutazone: used as a treatment for arthritis.

Chloramphenicol: Used for typhoid fever, and may contribute to bone-marrow depression, and/or leukemia.

Diphenylhydantoin: Used in treatment of epilepsy, and carries some risk of lymphomas.

Reserpine: Although a dispute arose in the mid-1970s that reserpine, used widely as a treatment for hypertension, increased the incidence of breast cancer, it has now been found that there is no association between this drug and breast cancer. Lab evidence shows increases in breast cancer in mice, but recent human studies have not supported the finding.

Amphetamines: Increases risk of lymphoma.

Opium: Addiction has been found to increase a person's susceptibility to develop esophageal and bladder cancer, presumably because of opium's tar content.

Iron Dextrose Complex: Soft tissue sarcomas have been found at the site of these injections.

CHAPTER SEVEN NOTES

1. Raven, R.W. *Cancer.* Vol. 1, London Butterworth, 1957

2. John Berg, "Can Nutrition Explain the International Epidemiology of Hormone Dependent Cancers?" *Cancer Research,* (Nov. 1975)

3. Berry Goldin, et. al., "Estrogen Excretion Pattern and Plasma Level in Vegetarian Women and Omnivorous Women," *New England Journal of Medicine,* (Dec. 1982)

4. Flora Rubin, et.al., *American Journal of Epidemiology,* (1985)

5. Blair Sabol, *The Body of America,* (New York: Arbor House, 1986)

6. *New England Journal of Medicine,* (Aug. 14, 1986)

7. Epstein, *Politics of Cancer.*

8. *New England Journal of Medicine,* (Aug. 14, 1960)

9. *Ibid.*

10. *Ibid.*

11. B. Hulka, et.al., *Journal of the American Medical Association,* (Jan. 22, 1982)

12. Cancer and Steroid Hormone Study, *New England Journal of Medicine,* (March 1987)

13. Elizabeth Holly; Noel S. Weiss; Jonathan I. List, "Cutaneous Melanoma in Relation to Exogenous Hormones and the Productive Factors," *Journal of the National Cancer Institute,* Vol. 70, #5. (May 1983)

14. James Neuberger, et. al. *The Lancet,* (Feb. 9, 1980)

15. Paul C. MacDonald, "Estrogen Plus Progestin in Postmenopausal Women," *New England Journal of Medicine,* (Dec. 31, 1981)

16. Muriel Standeven, et.al., "Change in Post Menopausal Estrogen Use," *American Journal of Epidemiology,* Vol. 124, #2. (1986)

17. Louise Brinton, et.al., "Menopausal Estrogen Use and Risk of Breast Cancer," *Cancer Journal of the American Cancer Society,* (May 15, 1981)

18. R. Don Gambrell, Jr., *Drug Therapy,* (Jan.1987)

19. Robert Meyers, *DES — The Bitter Pill,* (Seaview/Putnam: 1983)

20. W.J. Dieckman, et.al., *American Journal of Obstetrics and Gynecology,* (1953)

21. S. Robboy, et.al. Natl. Collaborative Diethylstilbestrol Adenosis Project. *Journal of the American Medical Association,* (Dec. 7, 1984)

22. Frank J. Leary, et.al., Mayo Clinic and Mayo Foundation, *Journal of the American Medical Association,* (Dec. 7, 1984)

23. Kenneth Kashkin, and Herbert Kleber, *Journal of the American Medical Association,* (Dec.8, 1989)

24. William E. Buckley, et al., "Estimated Prevalence of Anabolic Steroid Use Among Male High School Seniors," *Journal of American Medical Association,* (Dec. 16, 1988)

25. T. Thomas Taylor, and Adelbert E. Wade, *American Journal of Hospital Pharmacy,* (Sept. 1984)

26. Diane Young, and George P. Canellos, *Medical Clinics of North American,* (Nov. 1985)

27. Anna Meadows, and Jeffery Silber, *Ca-A Cancer Journal for Clinicians,* (Sept/Oct. 1985)

28. *Ibid.*

29. *Medical World News,* (Jan. 9, 1984)

30. Priscilla A. Gilman, and Neil Holtzman, *Journal of the American Medical Association.* (July 23, 1982)

31. Robert Stern, et.al., *New England Journal of Medicine,* (April 12, 1979)

32. J. Piper, *New England Journal of Medicine,* (Aug. 1, 1985)

33. *Cancer Epidemiology and Prevention.*

CHAPTER EIGHT

CONTAGIOUS CANCERS
AND THE IMMUNE SYSTEM

The case of David, the "Bubble Boy" who walked around in a NASA space suit, gave mass-media dramatization to the importance of a healthy immune system. David lived in a plastic bubble for 12 years because he had no viable immune system. He died ultimately of lymphatic cancer caused by an Epstein-Barr virus infection contracted after a bone marrow transplant from his own brother.

David's brief life provided research scientists and physicians with much more than dramatic press coverage. By studying David and observing him in his highly restricted, germ-free world, they were able to establish for certain the connection between viruses and cancer. He suffered from a hereditary deficiency of the immune system called Severe Combined Immune Deficiency (SCID), meaning that both parts of the immune system were deficient at birth. In general, patients with a deficient immune system have a 10,000 times greater risk of developing cancer compared to the general population.[1]

Fortunately, most of us have a fairly competent immune system. Even though we live in a sea of toxic agents in the air we breathe, the water we drink, the food we eat, and are exposed to radiation and all kinds of infections, our immune system guards us against them fairly efficiently.

157

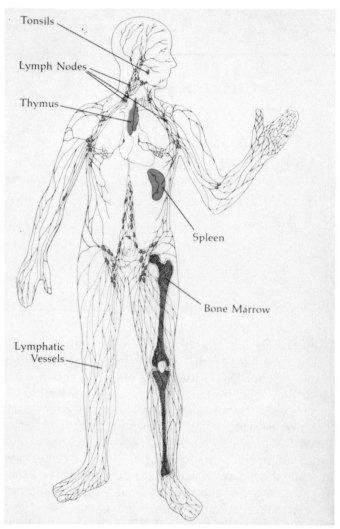

Tonsils

Lymph Nodes

Thymus

Spleen

Bone Marrow

Lymphatic
Vessels

The immune system consists of a number of cell types, including lymphocytes, plasma cells, macrophages, and granulocytes, as well as antibody molecules secreted by plasma cells. The cells are distributed throughout most of the body tissues, to which they are delivered by the bloodstream, but are concentrated in some areas.

Reprinted by permission, Scientific American *Medicine,* Section 6, Subsection I, ©1989, Scientific American, Inc. All rights reserved.

The immune system is the defense system of the body. It is made up of organs and cells. The primary organs for the immune system are bone marrow and the thymus gland. Bone marrow is the main factory where all the cells in the blood are manufactured and released into the blood stream. There are secondary organs of the immune system such as tonsils, adenoids, spleen, appendix and lymph nodes which are spread all over the body.

The bone marrow manufactures white blood cells, red blood cells and platelets. One group of white blood cells is called the lymphocytes. They are released directly into the blood stream and mature into B-cells and plasma cells. Some of the lymphocytes from the bone marrow go into the thymus gland for special training. They are called T-cells. The T-cells and B-cells constitute the two components of the immune system, both of which were missing in David.

These two components have entirely different functions. B-cells produce proteins or immunoglobulins which fight off infections. T-cells are involved in direct hand-to-hand combat with infectious agents. This second arm of the immune system, the T-cells, has gotten a lot of media attention lately because one category, called T4 or helper cells, is the type infected by the HIV virus. (The other two types of T-Cells are T8 and natural killer cells.) T4 cells are the master conductors of the human immune system orchestra. When these cells get infected with the HIV virus, the whole immune system goes out of order, causing AIDS patients to die with unusual and fulminating infections.

The human immune system can be deficient either at birth or becomes deficient from a serious infection, as in the case of the HIV virus leading to AIDS. There are other infectious agents like Hepatitis B, HPV or EBV (Epstein-Barr Virus) that can infect the body, and after a fist fight with the immune system, get a strong foothold in a particular organ and cause cancer. The strength of the immune system is important here in its ability to ward off such infections.

Good nutrition and exercise, a positive attitude, avoiding such things as tobacco smoke, alcohol's toxic chemicals and different sources of radiation, are very important in maintaining the viability of the immune system. Best news of all, cancer vaccines have been developed, medications that will boost our immune system to a point of wiping out cancer from the body altogether.

The power of a positive attitude and the ability to handle stress are emerging as strong factors in strengthening the immune system. We will deal with each one of these factors in detail in subsequent sections.

INFECTIONS

It is terrifying to imagine that cancer could be a contagious disease. Yet, there has been much evidence over the years, in observation of animals and humans, that this may be the case. We are exposed to many infections in our every-day lives that are caused by viruses, bacteria, and parasites. The nature of this public health problem is serious; viral infections are the most common cause of cancer world-wide. It is estimated that ten to 20 percent of the cancers in the western world and a higher percentage of cancers in Asia and Africa are caused by viruses.[2]

Among the viral infections that affect the immune system, the most notorious is Human Immune Deficiency Virus (HIV) that is known to cause AIDS. Then there are other viral infections like the Epstein-Barr Virus which can lead to lymphatic cancers, as in the case of the Bubble Boy, David. Hepatitis-B virus causes liver cancer in Africa and Asia. Human Papilloma virus infection causes warts on genitalia and areas of the mouth, which is seen commonly in AIDS patients, and may cause skin, oral and genital cancers as well. Another virus called HTLV-I causes leukemia in the United States, the Caribbean and Japan.

Parasitic infections like malaria, which is seen in tropical countries such as Asia and Africa, can also suppress the immune system. In Africa, there is a high incidence of lymphatic cancer called Burkitt's lymphoma, first described by Dr. Dennis Burkitt, caused by Epstein-Barr Virus Infection.

Historically speaking, scientists had begun to suspect by the early 1900s that cancer might be contagious, based on observations of pets and farm animals. In 1911, Peyton Rous, a research scientist in New York, demonstrated that a cancer in chickens could be experimentally transmitted to other chickens. This was followed by many similar experiments in other animals. In 1951, it was demonstrated that mouse leukemia was caused by a transmissible virus, and a similar laboratory proof was made for transmission of feline leukemia.

These findings inspired serious research for a virus-cancer connection in human beings. At our current level of understanding, cancer arises from a number of insults to the DNA, the master molecule of life. Viruses are one means of insult that can start the process rolling. A number of viruses have been isolated in humans which cause persistent infections that may lead to cancer. For example, Hepatitis-B virus can cause liver cancer, Genital Wart virus may cause genital cancer, and the Epstein-Barr virus that causes mononucleosis is the same virus that causes Burkitt Lymphoma in Africa and a throat cancer and thymic lymphomas in Asian countries.

160

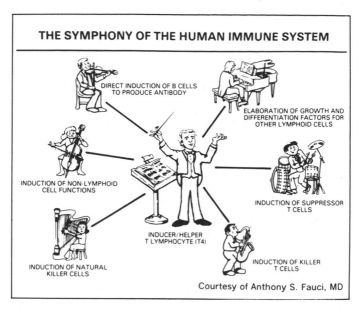

THE SYMPHONY OF THE HUMAN IMMUNE SYSTEM

DIRECT INDUCTION OF B CELLS
TO PRODUCE ANTIBODY

ELABORATION OF GROWTH AND
DIFFERENTIATION FACTORS FOR
OTHER LYMPHOID CELLS

INDUCTION OF NON-LYMPHOID
CELL FUNCTIONS

INDUCTION OF SUPPRESSOR
T CELLS

INDUCER/HELPER
T LYMPHOCYTE (T4)

INDUCTION OF NATURAL
KILLER CELLS

INDUCTION OF KILLER
T CELLS

Courtesy of Anthony S. Fauci, MD

Reprinted courtesy of Anthony S. Fauci, M.D.

These viruses are widespread, and many of us are exposed to them. Why don't we all get cancer from them? It is estimated that eighty percent of the United States population is infected with the Epstein-Barr virus. Why does only a very small percentage ever develop the related cancers from this virus?

The answer is found in the human immune system and its function as a protector of the human body. If the immune system is compromised by other infections, immunosuppressive drugs, poor nutrition, or damaged by toxic chemicals, these viruses are not kept under check any more and can flare up to cause cancer. As we see in the recent epidemic of AIDS, those who are stricken may get many cancers caused by the virus that has invaded their bodies, like genital wart virus causing cancers in the mouth and anal area. There is high suspicion that cytomegalovirus (CMV) causes Kaposi's Sarcoma. Significant progress has already been made in the area of control of these viral diseases by vaccines, as in the case of feline leukemia virus vaccine which was released in 1985, but there is still a long way to go.

VIRUSES: NATURE'S 'PERFECT' PARASITES

The virus is the most extreme form of parasite. It lacks the cell structures common to all forms of life. A virus does not need and cannot metabolize nutrients. It also cannot replicate without the help of its host.

161

The popular video game Pac-Man gives a good visual comparison to the activity that goes on within the cells of the human body when attacked by a virus. This invader is actually much smaller than the gobbling video creation, a mere 1/16,000th the size of the head of a pin, but just as voracious. Some viruses, like those producing the common cold, look like soccer balls. The flu virus looks like the head of a Roman mace, and herpes and AIDS viruses are spherical. By whatever shape, they are all admirable in their streamlined, minimalist design, consisting simply of a core of genetic material which is either a DNA or an RNA molecule and a protective envelope made of proteins. Dr. Steven Straus of the National Institute of Health (NIH) remarked that there is no waste in a virus; every piece is there for a reason, and that is what makes it a magnificent little structure.

RETROVIRUSES

Retroviruses are a special class of molecular pirates. "Retro" means reverse, which in terms of these viruses implies reverse flow of genetic information from RNA to DNA instead of the normal flow from DNA to RNA. They have this ability from an enzyme called reverse transcriptase.

There are two families of viruses in this broad group—HIV and HTLV. Both groups have two subgroups each, HIV into HIV-1 and 2, and HTLV into HTLV-1 and -2. HIV-1 causes AIDS whereas HIV-2 causes a milder illness.

HTLV-1 is a distant cousin to HIV-1. It was the first virus to be discovered in the retrovirus families and was first reported in the United States in 1980. It has been found in epidemic proportions in some "hot spots" around the world, like southwest Japan, the Caribbean and Africa. This virus can be transmitted from mother to child during pregnancy and breast feeding. It is also transmitted by sexual intercourse and sharing of contaminated needles. Presently one to two million people are affected with HTLV-1. Out of the infected, one in 1,500 is at risk of developing a rare cancer called Acute T-cell Lymphoma/Leukemia (ATL), a type of leukemia.[3] There has been up to a 30 percent increase of the development of ATL in drug abusers and blacks in southeastern United States.

HTLV-1 can cause lymphatic cancer in the skin and ATL. Prevention is similar to the steps we take for AIDS prevention discussed later in this chapter. Currently, all blood used for transfusions is screened for HTLV-1.

HTLV-2 causes some cases of hairy cell leukemia and other lymphatic cancers.

Viruses in both families, HIV and HTLV, are transmitted in the same manner. Risk factors are also the same: they can be spread through blood exchange, sexual intercourse, and from mother to child. The preventive strategies are also similar.

As with all viruses, public education is necessary for reducing infection by preventing transmission. Screening techniques of blood transfusions are a step in the right direction, but eventually a vaccine must be developed.

AIDS: A Contemporary Epidemic

In 1981, the Centers for Disease Control in Atlanta, Georgia, came across some unsettling reports. There were several cases of a form of Kaposi's Sarcoma reported in New York and California that was proving fatal to its victims. All persons stricken were male, young to middle aged, and gay.

Why puzzling? Kaposi's Sarcoma was a cancer that had first been described in 1872 by Kaposi, a Hungarian dermatologist. Although Kaposi described it as "lethal," modern physicians and scientists had never determined it to be "aggressive." By 1950, there were only 600 cases of Kaposi's Sarcoma recorded in the entire world literature on cancer, and annual cancer statistics indicated that a mere three people out of one million might develop Kaposi's Sarcoma in their lifetimes.

Physicians saw the disease infrequently, usually in elderly men. They began thinking of it as a rare, less threatening, indolent type of skin cancer. It had become an odd, bizarre occurrence to be studied primarily by pathologists and dermatologists.

Slowly more information began to accumulate at the Atlanta Centers for Disease Control. In 1981 a few more cases appeared, this time among heterosexuals who were intravenous drug abusers, and by 1982 there were more reports in hemophiliacs who received frequent blood transfusions. The reports included cases of Kaposi's Sarcoma and other cancers, with descriptions of other seldom-seen infections arising from a compromised immune system — such as pneumocystis carinii pneumonia (caused by a parasite which infiltrates the lung tissue). Physicians commonly refer to a spectrum of seemingly unrelated diseases such as these a "syndrome."

There seemed to be no explanation for the reported cases, and what was worse, no cure. The patients in question had been healthy, but were suddenly weakened and riddled with horrible diseases which confounded textbook explanations. Their conditions defied chemotherapy, antibiotics, cortisone and immunosuppressive drugs. Similar to Kaposi's description of the disease in a much different era—with a much more limited scientific understanding—the current disease was lethal within two to three years, and sometimes even sooner. Auto-Immune Deficiency Syndrome (AIDS), and all of its physical, emotional and economic misery had entered the American consciousness.

Through the Looking Glass

Groups of persons considered at highest risk in the United States for AIDS are: male homosexuals, intravenous drug abusers, Haitian refugees, hemophiliacs, infants receiving blood transfusions, female sexual partners of males with AIDS, male prison inmates, and female prostitutes. Now all adults are at risk because heterosexual transmission of AIDS has become more prevalent.

There are three phases of HIV infection:[4]

1. Acute Phase or Early Phase: flu-like symptoms lasting weeks,
2. Middle or Chronic Phase: lasts years, may or may not have symptoms,
3. Final or Crisis Phase: what we call AIDS-related complex or AIDS. This lasts months to years.

The most common symptoms to watch in the Crisis Phase are:

1. Swollen lymph glands or "nodes";
2. Persistent fatigue;
3. Fevers and night sweats;
4. Weight loss;
5. Diarrhea; and
6. Thrush in the mouth and difficulty swallowing.

These symptoms can all be indicative of many illnesses, including emotional disorders such as depression. A physician must therefore ask the right questions and probe further. A routine blood test will indicate a healthy or a weakened immune system. To make a more specific diagnosis of Kaposi's Sarcoma (which occurs in a small percentage of those patients suffering from AIDS), a physician must perform a tissue biopsy on one of the reddish patches or lumps.

The origin of HIV virus appears to be uncertain but it appears the virus started in Africa and silently spread in the mid to late 1970s. AIDS was discovered in 1981 and the HIV virus in 1983. Diagnostic testing for the virus has much improved since 1985, and we now have a fairly clear picture of the extent and distribution of this worldwide problem.

The World Health Organization maintains an international surveillance of AIDS called the "Global Program on AIDS." As of October, 1989, 100,410 cases of AIDS were reported worldwide. Estimates of the actual count are much higher because of the possibility of underreporting; it is possible that as many as five to ten million people are infected worldwide with the HIV-1 virus.[5]

DID YOU KNOW THAT?

- According to the Centers for Disease Control in Atlanta, from 1981 to 1989 there have been approximately 100,000 cases of AIDS reported and 59,000 AIDS related deaths.
- The first 50,000 cases of AIDS were reported from 1981 to 1987 and second 50,000 cases from 1987 to 1989.
- By 1991, the United States Public Health Service predicts that there will be 270,000 cases of AIDS in the United States and 179,000 fatalities, making it one of the nation's top ten killers.
- Presently there are one to 1.5 million people infected with HIV-1 in the United States. Of these, 54 percent will develop AIDS in ten years and 99 percent will eventually develop AIDS.
- By 1991, medical economists predict that AIDS will add 1.4 percent to the annual United States health care budget, or 10.9 billion dollars a year, assuming that the expense of caring for each AIDS patient will be no more than 50,000 dollars per year.
- By 1991, the prevalence of AIDS in the heterosexual population will increase from its present seven percent to nine percent.

Prevention for HIV/AIDS

Acquired Immune Deficiency virus appears to be transmitted through three routes: sexual contact, blood and blood products, and pregnancy. There are some steps that can be taken for prevention in these three areas.[6]

For preventing sexual transmission of the virus, either abstinence or having a safe, uninfected partner is the most important factor. The greater the number of sexual partners the greater the risk of contracting AIDS. Indiscriminate sexual activity puts all people at risk, regardless of sexual preference. An HIV infected person will develop antibodies to the virus in three months which are detectable by a blood test. Preferably, a couple should know the results of blood tests before they decide to be sexually active. Testing is almost 100 percent accurate these days.

1. Since sexual abstinence is often out of the question, we are left with the choice of "safe sex." A decrease in the number of sexual partners is important. If sexual contact is not within a

long term monogamous relationship, where neither partner is infected, use of double protection—condom with spermicide—for each occasion and with all kinds of sexual activity. If one partner is infected, the chance of the other becoming infected is 10-70 percent. Male to female transmission of the infection appears to be more efficient than vice versa.

2. Since 1985, standard testing of blood for AIDS is required in all blood banks throughout the world, making blood and blood products much safer now. A recent trend in surgical procedures has been to encourage patients to donate blood for their own transfusions during surgery — called autologous transfusions.

3. The main message for drug abusers is: "Don't share needles." Although society does not condone drug abuse, in this case it must choose the lesser of two evils. Needles can be disinfected with undiluted bleach, a cheap and apparently effective method of sterilization. The needle must be flushed out completely before self-injection with a shared syringe.

    Intravenous drug abusers who share needles generally run a 10-80 percent risk of becoming HIV infected through tainted blood on the needles.[7] These abusers, at high risk of contracting AIDS, are being helped through drug rehabilitation programs and through needle exchange programs which exist in many cities, providing free sterilized needles.

4. It should be mandatory that pregnant women be tested for possible HIV infection. The risk of fetal infection in a pregnant woman with AIDS is about 30-40 percent.

HIV-2 is a close cousin to HIV-1, but causes a milder infection and is quite rare in the United States. This was first described in 1985 in African prostitutes and later in African AIDS patients. In 1987 a West African woman in the United States was reported to have HIV-2, and since then a few more cases have been reported. Since the mode of transmission of this virus is similar to HIV-1, preventive steps are basically the same.

HEPATITIS-B: A SILENT SLEEPER

One day in July, 1984, an Intensive Care nurse at a Hospital in Ann Arbor, Michigan, was diagnosed as having acute Hepatitis-B infection. She had mild, flu-like symptoms. Within a few weeks three more nurses and a resident at the same hospital were diagnosed with the same illness. None of them appeared terribly ill, and four of the stricken individuals recovered uneventfully. However, one died. These people had caught the hepatitis virus at work.[8]

Compared to other countries, the United States has a low incidence of the Hepatitis-B virus. Still, 200,000 Americans are infected with this virus each year. Out of this number 50,000 have a mild infection, and another 10,000 develop a serious illness. Ten thousand more become chronic carriers who are not sick themselves but can transmit the infection to others. This is similar to the "Typhoid Mary" phenomenon at the turn of the century, when a food handler passed a typhoid fever that she had contacted onto hundreds of people but never became sick herself.

Current estimates state that there are 400,000 to 800,000 carriers of Hepatitis-B in the United States. Alaskan Eskimos have a very high incidence of this disease in comparison to the rest of the United States.[9] Worldwide, there is a different picture. There are more than 200 million carriers of the disease, particularly in Africa, the Mediterranean basin, the Middle East, the South Sahara in Africa, Southeast Asia, China and Japan.

The most serious consequence of Hepatitis-B infection is that it has been found to be a cause of liver cancer. While it causes only three cases per 100,000 deaths in the United States and Western Europe, it is responsible for 25 to 100 cases per 100,000 deaths in the above-mentioned high risk areas of the world, making liver cancer the leading cause of all deaths.[10]

The Hepatitis-B virus can be found in all bodily secretions, but the heaviest concentration is in the blood, semen and vaginal fluid. Thus, the virus can be transmitted through exchange of bodily secretions and blood.

The virus is often transmitted through blood in occupational contact, such as the example of the health workers in Ann Arbor. Blood transfusions used to be a common mode of transmission before 1970 when routine testing for Hepatitis-B began. Once again, IV drug abusers are at very high risk for catching this disease through use of contaminated needles.

Right now, sexual contact is the most common mode of transmission of this virus, with the transfer of infection much like that of the HIV. Bisexual men, IV drug abusers and other carriers give the infection to their sexual partners.

During pregnancy, the Hepatitis-B can be transmitted to the fetus. Ninety percent of infants born to pregnant Hepatitis-B carrier women get infected with Hepatitis-B and 80-90 percent become chronic carriers.[11]

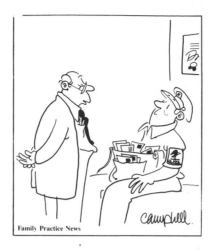

"You're perfectly healthy, but
you're a carrier."

Reprinted from Family Practice News, January 15-31, 1985,
●1985, Fairchild Publications, a division of Capital Cities
Media, Inc., and Ms. Martha F. Campbell.

Casual contact within families that have poor hygiene has caused an increased incidence of the disease among siblings.

Many studies around the world have shown that this virus can cause cancer in both humans and in animals. In a carefully conducted experiment at the University of California, woodchucks were exposed to Hepatitis-B virus. Ninety percent of those animals that had chronic active hepatitis developed liver cancer.

Prevention for Hepatitis-B

The hepatitis vaccine is available in two forms, called Heptavax and Energix B. The United States Public Health Services Advisory Committee on Immunization Practices (ACIP) recommends the following groups for vaccinations:[12]

1. Health care workers and morticians, especially those at risk for exposure to blood and blood products;
2. Persons at high risk of needle stick injuries such as doctors, nurses, dentists, lab technicians, etc.;

168

3. High risk persons such as homosexually active males or sexually active heterosexuals, IV drug abusers or hemophiliacs;
4. Patients and staff in hemodialysis units;
5. Mentally retarded persons and any staff taking care of them;
6. Inmates of long term correctional facilities;
7. The household and sexual contacts of Hepatitis-B carriers;
8. The newborns of Hepatitis-B carriers should receive gamma globulin and Hepatitis-B vaccine (all pregnant women should be screened for Hepatitis-B virus in their first prenatal visit);
9. Special high risk groups in the United States such as Alaskan Eskimos, native Pacific Islanders, and immigrants and refugees from Asia and Africa; and
10. Americans who travel abroad.

Carriers of Hepatitis-B Virus

Carriers should be screened periodically for Alpha Feto Protein (AFP) levels, a blood test for a protein released by the liver cancer. It is routinely done in the United States' Eskimo populations because of high incidence of Hepatitis-B carrier rate and liver cancer. Another hepatitis virus called Hepatitis-C transmitted by blood transfusions has been linked to liver cancer, according to recent reports.

HUMAN PAPILLOMA VIRUS — THE BED BUG

The human papilloma virus "bed bug" is responsible for the new sexual plague affecting society. AIDS, syphilis, herpes, gonorrhea, chlamydia—and infections caused by the Human Papilloma Virus (HPV)—are all well known sexually transmitted diseases. Combined, it is estimated that every American aged 15-55 will catch a sexually transmitted disease at some point in his or her life, and there are approximately 270,000 new cases of sexually transmitted diseases seen every day. One million Americans are infected with HPV every year.[13] According to the Department of Health and Human Services, an estimate of total cases of human papilloma virus in 1988 were ten to 12 million.

There are 56 different types of papilloma viruses that can infect humans and a wide range of animals including horses, cattle, and birds say Drs. Ralph Richart and Kenneth Trofatter. The most common manifestation of this virus is the simple plantar wart. A few of other papilloma viruses are responsible for genital warts, and two of the 56 have been consistently present in cervical cancers and cervical dysplasia, an abnormal cell change that precedes cancer of the cervix. Sexual transmission from the asymptomatic condylomas of the penis occurs frequently.[14] Cervical cancer kills approximately 6,800 women each year in the United States, and approximately 500,000 cases of cervical cancer are reported annually worldwide.

Advances in molecular biology and genetic engineering over the past decade have shed new light on the ubiquitous, annoying skin tags caused by the papilloma virus, and robbed some of them of their innocence. By the late 1970s scientists were able to examine tissue taken from cervical cancer patients and actually look for traces as small as viruses. What was the result of these microscopic investigations? The papilloma virus was contained in 90 percent of the cervical cancers sampled!

Papilloma virus is also turning up in microscopic examination of 90 percent of cervical dysplasias, in cancers of the vagina and vulva, and in cancer of the penis. There is an unfortunate revelation from this finding: papilloma lesions have been found in the genital region of young female children — increasingly thought to be a telltale sign of sexual molestation.

Children can be infected in the larynx (voice box) from the mother at the time of delivery, which causes wart growths on the vocal cords called laryngeal papillomas. Other infections caused by the human papilloma virus in men may eventually lead to penile cancer. Anal cancers related to HPV have also been seen in AIDS patients.[15]

It appears that the entire lower genital tract is susceptible to papilloma infection. About 500,000 women each year are now seeking treatment for genital warts, an increase of 500 percent over the past 20 years. The peak incidence is in women aged 20 to 24 years old.[16] Multiple sex partners and early age of intercourse are causes. This infection and the resulting cancer are not seen in celibate women.

The presence of a papilloma virus infection in a woman's male partner is a greater risk to her than her own sexual behavior. Men with genital warts put their female partners at high risk for cancer. Philandering husbands are dangerous to the health of their wives, because they can acquire cancer-causing viruses through sexual contact and pass this agent on to their wives. Dr. I. Martinez studied Puerto Ricans, and found that wives of men with penile cancer were at high risk for cervical cancer.[17] A study done at the University of Oxford by a team of investigators showed that wives of husbands with more than 15 partners were at eight times the risk for precancerous conditions (cervical dysplasia carcinoma in situ or cervical cancer).[18] A recent study done by Dr. Renzo Barrasso and associates in Paris showed that husbands of the women with precancerous or cancerous conditions of the cervix also showed HPV infections. The genital warts were seen in 309 of the 480 men examined—a clear indication that it is a sexually transmitted disease.[19]

The virus does not act alone but needs a co-factor—cigarette smoking, malnutrition with vitamin deficiency, and so forth—to have an effect. In laboratory experiments with cottontail rabbits, the virus causes warts that sometimes develop into malignant tumors, but the progression occurs much more frequently and rapidly if coal tar with a multitude of carcinogens are applied to the warts.[20] In humans, smoking has been implicated as such a co-factor. Women who smoke have a four times greater risk of developing cervical cancer in their lifetimes. Additional co-factors are genetic or acquired immune deficiency, other genital infections such as herpes, ultraviolet light and other agents toxic to the immune system. Deficiency of vitamin C and vitamin A have also been implicated. Recent reports show that HPV is the cause of many cancers, including those of the male/female genitalia, the skin around the fingers, cancers around the eyelids and oral and anal cancers.[21]

Prevention for Papilloma Virus

For the future, researchers have found a diagnostic test similar to a Pap smear to determine which type of papilloma virus may be present. It is called ViraPap and is manufactured by Life Technologies in Maryland.

A vaccine to ward off the initial infection would be a major step, and a biotechnology firm in Minnesota is having initial success with such a vaccine for cattle.

Currently, the best methods of prevention appear to be use of condoms during intercourse, annual Pap smears and a colposcopy exam (use of magnification for visual examination of the vagina). Pap smears are helpful in detecting the disease, but not always foolproof, for the virus can hide in normal looking cells. Studies at Georgetown University show that out of a substantial number of women with cervical papilloma virus, between five to ten percent have normal Pap smears. Colposcopy has been found to be very helpful in early detection of precancerous changes and cancer of the female reproductive tract.

Kits are now available to physicians to type HPV in the genital warts (such as the ViraPap mentioned earlier). Of the 56 different types of HPV warts, types 16 and 18 are the most dangerous. Types 31, 33, 35, 52-56 are considered of moderate risk and types 6 and 11 rarely cause malignancy.

EPSTEIN-BARR VIRUS — THE "KISSING DISEASE"

The Epstein-Barr Virus (EBV) is named after two scientists, Epstein and Barr, who discovered the virus in 1964. The virus appears to be a sexually transmitted disease. Studies done in Denmark, Scotland, the United States and Sweden in the 1970s indicated that individuals stricken with "mono" have almost a six times greater chance than the general population of developing Hodgkin's Disease after a lapse of three to 13 years.[22]

Epstein-Barr Virus, one of the herpes viruses, has been isolated as a cause for Burkitt's Lymphoma, a lymphatic cancer that strikes children in Africa, a throat cancer called Nasopharyngeal Carcinoma which is common in Asia, as well as "mono" in western countries. The nickname, "the kissing disease" is appropriate for describing mononucleosis. It is highly contagious, most prevalent among teenagers and young adult men and women, and generally spread through saliva like a common cold. It can be diagnosed when EBV specific antibodies show up in serum and blood tests early after the onset of the disease. These antibody concentrations decline during convalescence but remain detectable throughout life, providing an immunity to the disease. However, these same elevated antibodies affecting EBV show up in many patients with Hodgkin's disease. In fact, clusters of Hodgkin's disease have appeared in school populations that have had outbreaks of mono.[23]

Does the EBV cause human cancer? Or does it merely colonize malignant cells that have already been transformed by other means? One thing that scientists have been able to demonstrate is that the human lymphocytic response to the EBV is extraordinary. This virus stimulates repeated rounds of cell division in B-Cell lymphocytes because they possess a receptor for the EBV virus on their surfaces.

Prevention for the Epstein-Barr Virus

One manner of prevention of the Epstein-Barr virus is simply by improving hygiene by decreasing the exchange of saliva, especially on toys contaminated with saliva. As with other viruses, there is a possibility of vaccine in the future, and a vaccine has been found which protects animals.[24] Until such a discovery, then, high risk individuals, those who have chronic mono infections in particular, should be followed carefully for cancer.

Malaria is very common in Africa, and malarial types of infection appear to be a co-factor in Epstein-Barr virus.

OTHER INFECTIONS

Viruses are not the only ones that cause contagious diseases that have an association with cancer. Certain chronic bacterial and parasitic infections can predispose people to cancer, as well as certain chronic inflammatory diseases which are suspected to put certain people at

172

higher risk for cancer. Some people who have chronic skin ulcers are at risk for skin cancer.[25]

In Egypt, most of the rivers and ponds are infested with a parasite called bladder fluke. This parasite is responsible for high rates of bladder infection due to bathing and swimming in infested water, eventually leading to bladder cancer (Schistosomiasis). The best preventative is to towel dry completely so that parasites will not be able to get into the body.[26]

In Asia, liver fluke—another parasite like bladder fluke and also transmitted through contaminated water—is a very common infection. Liver fluke can cause a high incidence of biliary tract cancer where the parasite commonly resides and causes irritation.

Inflammatory Bowel Diseases: Ulcerative Colitis and Crohn's Disease

Patients with these diseases are at high risk for bowel cancer if the disease is extensive and has been experienced for more than 10-15 years. The risk for bowel cancer appears to be five to ten times higher in people with ulcerative colitis than for people without.[27]

Crohn's disease, on the other hand, may give rise to increased risk of colon cancer up to 20 times as high as the risk for the non-diseased population.[28]

THE IMMUNE SYSTEM

Immunosuppressive Drugs

As discussed in the opening part of this chapter, infectious agents and chance combinations of heredity immune system deficiency are not the only causes for a suppression of the immune system. Man-made biotechnology can also be to blame. Anti-rejection, immunosuppressive drugs have been a major breakthrough in enabling surgeons to perform successful transplant operations. To make the transplanted organ more acceptable to the body and reduce the risks of these patients' immune systems rejecting the transplanted organ, patients are given high doses of anti-rejection, immunosuppressive drugs. This creates a see-saw effect, for when you raise one end, the other end is lowered. Anti-rejection drugs make the organ acceptable by suppressing the immune system, but they impair the body's ability to resist infections. Thus infections will rage unchecked in an immunodeficient body. Infections can be so fulminant that they can produce lymphatic cancers called lymphomas as early as six months after a transplant operation. These patients have a 100 times increased risk of developing cancer.[29] The common drugs used in this category are cyclophosphamide, azathioprine (cyclosporin A), and corticosteroids.

Kidney transplant patients have shown a 30-60 times increase in risk of a lymphatic cancer called non-Hodgkin's Lymphoma.[30]

Other cancers seen in transplant patients are skin cancer, leukemias, thyroid cancer, lung cancer and Kaposi's Sarcoma.[31] Skin cancer is seen four times more in transplant patients, and these patients have an eight times increased risk of malignancy in the cervix.[32]

In AIDS patients and other immunosuppressed patients, it is suspected that Epstein Barr virus goes unchecked and causes brain Lymphomas.[33]

Immunosuppressive drugs like corticosteroids have also been used therapeutically for treating many other diseases like severe rheumatoid arthritis, chronic nephritis (inflammation of the kidney) and lupus. Patients with connective tissue disease, once their immune systems are compromised, have similar risks for getting cancer.

Many cancer patients have a depressed immune system anyway, which becomes further suppressed when chemotherapeutic agents or radiation therapy are used, leaving them at higher risk for developing cancer.

Tobacco and Marijuana

The chemicals in tobacco and marijuana smoke have many poisons that suppress the immune system. Adult smokers and children exposed to second hand smoke get upper respiratory tract infections two-and-a-half times more often than the non-smoking population. They suffer from bronchitis more often, and have a higher incidence of ear infections. (*See also* Chapter 3 on Tobacco) Peggy Mann, in her book *Marijuana Alert*, writes that the cells of the immune system do not appear to function well against infection because the cells themselves are on a "high."[34]

Radiation

Radiation exposure in terms of sunlight or artificial ultraviolet light suppresses the cells of the immune system in the skin, as is evident from flare-ups of herpes upon exposure to sunlight or sunlamps. Laboratory experiments using both natural sunlight and sunlamps show depression of the immune system in the skin itself, as mentioned in Chapter 4 on sunlight. Large doses of radiation exposure to the entire body also suppresses the immune system.

Chemicals

Many industrial products used at the work place and at home are hazardous to the immune system. Some examples are: pesticides, formaldehyde, vinyl chloride from plastic and artificial rubber industries, and heavy metals such as lead, arsenic, cadmium, and mercury (which are common pollutants in air and water). Dioxin has a specific effect on the thymus gland, a principal organ of the immune system, leaving the body especially vulnerable to the toxic effects of dioxin. PCB and PBB also are very potent suppressors of the immune system, as shown in lab experiments with animals, and in humans.[35]

The Aging Immune System

One fact that has been consistently observed is that as we age, we are at greater risk for getting cancer. In fact, age is the most important risk factor for cancer. There are two explanations for this phenomenon. One is that, like other body tissues, the immune system weakens and wears out, as shown by the increased number of infections seen in the elderly. Sickness and deaths due to these infections are greater in the elderly than in young adults.[36] Thus, the immune system's ability to police the body, discern the new cancer cells that are forming and destroy them, is impaired. The cancer is able to get a foothold in a body that might otherwise be healthy and resistent to disease.

The second explanation for increased cancer rates among the elderly is that during our lifetimes we are repeatedly exposed to all kinds of environmental insults, such as tobacco smoke, radiation, sunlight, and chemicals which result in cellular mutations (as explained in the section on Biology). Cancer, then is the cumulative effect of all of these insults. It appears that the aging thymus gland, which starts shrinking at puberty to middle age, allows the increasing tendency for infectious cancers.

Stress, Emotions, Immune System and Cancer

"I don't get depressed, I just grow a tumor," said Woody Allen in 1982. In the past, death and taxes were the only sure things in life. But now we can say with certainty that stress will be in our lives whether we like it or not. Stress has been named the disease of the 1980s, but I am sure it is going to be around for a long time to come, as it has been around from time immemorial. Its relationship to disease has been long suspected also. The Greek physician Galen, a disciple of Hippocrates, noted that "melancholy women" were at higher risk for developing cancers than "sanguine women."[37]

Even with the relationship between stress and disease a little more clear, all the evidence is not yet in. The immune system has a very important role in combating cancer, especially viral induced cancers. Most of the researchers feel that small cancers are forming in all of us regularly, and the immune system fights them off by policing the body. So far there is no conclusive relationship between stress and cancer.[38]

There are four elements involved in stress: the first is the stressful situation to which we are exposed; second is the type of personality we have; third is lifestyle factors, which are important in understanding how we perceive the stress; and fourth is adjustment, or how we cope with it.

Research on Stress

Stress appears to deplete the immune system. Animal research has shown that stress increases the size of transplanted or viral induced tumors by decreasing the number of natural killer cells of the immune system, according to a study by Dr. Vernon Riley.[39] In human beings, the response to stress has been studied in a number of ways. A study done on 64 dental students by psychologist John B. Jemmott, leading a team of researchers from Harvard and Tufts universities, showed a decrease of immunoglobulin A (IGA) levels before exams. IGA in saliva normally fights off viruses that cause colds. Those dental students who dealt with stress in a relaxed way had higher IGA levels.[40] The similar study on persons in the stressful position of caring for Alzheimer's disease patients, showed an impairment in the functioning of their immune system.[41]

Studies of patients with different mental conditions, such as depression, schizophrenia, or bereavement have been done to show a detrimental effect upon the immune system. Loss of a loved one is one of the most stressful events that can happen in a person's life, and the grief reaction that usually follows can be extremely stressful. In a "Broken-Heart" study done in 1969, Dr. C.M. Parkes and associates studied the increased death rate among widowers; in the first six months after the death of a spouse, half of them died of a heart attack.[42] Because depressive illnesses seem to cause alterations in immune functions, they are associated with increased risk for infection and also for cancer.[43]

The mechanism of stress, it appears, affects the brain, both directly through the nervous system and indirectly through the hormonal system.[44] We handle stress by increasing the circulating steroids, such as corticosteroids, secreted by the adrenal glands. The adrenal cortex is under control of the hormone ACTH from the anterior pituitary, which is in turn controlled by the hypothalamus in the brain—the ultimate seat of emotions. Similar conclusions were drawn in another study by Dr. Neil Graham and his colleagues of the University of South Australia.[45]

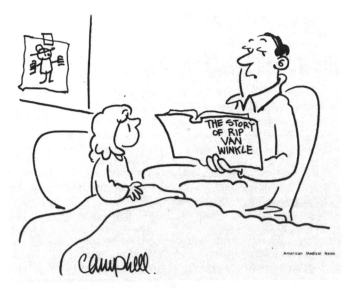

"Yes, he probably was a type B personality."

Reprinted from Family Practice News, Jan. 15-31, 1985, ©1985, Fairchild Publications, a division of Capital Cities Media, Inc., and from Ms. Martha F. Campbell.

Personality Factors and Stress

Personality factors are the second piece to this puzzle. Here, evidence is quite vague. It appears that the Type C personality—individuals who were distant from their parents physically or emotionally in childhood—tend to repress emotions during adult life. Naturally, they have difficulty in forming and sustaining relationships, and may not be able to cope with stress. The resulting impairment of their immune systems may make them less able to fight disease.[46]

Lifestyle Factors

When combining stress and personality, how does one perceive stress? Some stress may be good for us, making us competitive. It appears that stress is good as long as one knows things are under control, but becomes detrimental when it creates feelings of helplessness. The issue of lifestyle comes in here. A stressed person may begin smoking, drinking alcohol, not eat or sleep well, and not take care of himself or herself. Such a person may not use medical services wisely, either by avoiding them altogether or using them too much, becoming a hypochondriac. Stress at this level has created a person who is unable to cope with situations or his/her health.

Adjustment to Stress

An adjustment to the above problems is easier when there is a good social support system. People who have a good social network turn out to be good "copers," but for those who are socially isolated, coping becomes increasingly difficult.

How to make a good coper out of a poor coper? There are a number of ways. A regular exercise program or participation in sports is a good diversion. Hobbies such as painting, drawing or music can help. Having a pet is also helpful, and volunteering for a community activity will leave a person feeling better.

Relaxation techniques are available which deal with the coping mechanism and also boost the immune system. Meditation seems to help as well. Biofeedback is a technique of self-help taught in many places. I personally found the Biofeedback program at the Cleveland Clinic very useful. (For more information, contact: *Biofeedback Society of America, 4301 Owens Street, Wheatridge, Colorado, 80033.*) Visual imagery techniques appear to help some cancer patients in preventing a recurrence of the disease or to help cope with the present condition more positively. At present, research is underway for pharmacological intervention, but no drug is available yet.

There is one foolproof way for relaxation: humor. I believe that a motto in hospitals should be, "Humor is a hazard to your illness." All hospitals and health-care facilities should have laughing rooms where people can watch comedies or reruns of favorite television sitcom classics. We all can be a little more "laid back" without compromising our work ethic.

Diet and the Immune System

Because the immune system is primarily made up of cells and proteins, nutritional deficiencies will weaken it noticeably—as seen in malnourished patients. In severe cases of malnutrition, the abnormalities in the immune system are similar to those of AIDS patients.[47] High fat diets or excessive caloric intake impair the functioning of the immune system as well; for example, obese infants have more respiratory tract infections. Abusive use of alcohol also impairs the functions of the immune system, as mentioned in Chapter Six on Alcohol.

The proper amount of minerals (calcium, magnesium sulfate, and iodine) and vitamins is also necessary for optimal functioning of the immune system. Nobel-prize winner Dr. Linus Pauling spent a lifetime promoting the benefits of orange juice and vitamin C as a protection against colds for this reason. Now the ideal diet consists of balanced meals which are high in protein, low in fats, rich in minerals and vitamins, and little or no alcohol. Also important is avoiding contaminants such as aflatoxins, PCB, PBB, Agent Orange, pesticides, and polycyclic hydrocarbons from cigarette smoke. These steps should be coupled with a moderate amount of exercise.

Recently, some vitamins and minerals have been found to be very promising in stimulating the immune system in AIDS patients. For example, vitamin A, vitamin C and vitamin E have been shown to enhance the immune system. According to Dr. K.N. Prasad, a world famous authority on vitamins and trace minerals, vitamins prevent the promotional stage of cancer formation even though the exact mechanism of the process is not known. One of the important mechanisms by which vitamins reduce the risk of cancer is through stimulation of the immune system, as mentioned earlier. Some data of similar nature is being accumulated in human beings also.

Dr. J.D. Kanofsky and associates of the Albert Einstein School of Medicine found that vitamin A and beta-carotene repair the damage caused by trauma, malnutrition, infections, stress, radiation, and chemotherapy to the immune system of laboratory animals.[48] But here megadoses of vitamin A were used—about 10-15 times the recommended dietary allowance. Similar results have been seen in human beings, creating the general consensus among scientists that vitamin A is a stimulant to the immune system and may help AIDS patients.

Megadoses of vitamin E, up to 800 units daily (instead of the recommended daily allowance of 8-10 units), enhance the function of the key cells in the immune system, called T cells. Research done at Tufts University in Boston showed that they produce more of the chemical called interleukin-II, which enables the immune system to fight infections better.

Among the minerals, zinc seems to have a very important role in immune system functioning. Dr. Ananda Prasad, known internationally as "Dr. Zinc," has done much research on the mineral. He found that populations consuming a high cereal diet as in India may become zinc deficient due to interference in absorption of zinc in the gut. Zinc supplements may be advised for these populations. Dr. Lourdes Corman describes a study in which 15 institutionalized patients were given 220 mg. of zinc supplement daily for a month; they showed an improvement in their immune system functioning, checked by Tetanus shots.[49] Slightly zinc deficient Rhesus monkeys had trouble gaining weight and failed to thrive; their immune functions were depressed by 20-30 percent.[50]

Exercise and the Immune System

We have known for a long time that a moderate amount of exercise is good for our well being. But immunity appears to wear down with "intensive" exercise. For example, in a study of more than 1,800 marathoners in Los Angeles in 1987, it was shown that 13 percent became sick with colds and flu, compared to two percent of runners that were on the sidelines.[51] In contrast, a study by the Centers for Disease Control (CDC) in Atlanta found that an average jogger who exercised moderately, logging about 25 miles a week, showed a rate of 1.2 colds per athlete compared to three colds per person in the general population.

Professor Laurel McKinnon, a lecturer in exercise physiology and wellness at Australia's University of Queensland, confirmed other studies done on human beings and animals on the relationship between exercise and immunity. She felt that the intensity of exercise was critical: intense daily exercise reduces an athlete's resistance to infectious diseases, including colds and flu, while moderate exercise seems to improve the function of the immune system.[52]

Mild to moderate exercise, then, appears to strengthen our immune system.

IMMUNOTHERAPY AND SPONTANEOUS REMISSIONS

Immunotherapy is a way of stimulating and promoting the immune system as a whole or in part to prevent or control cancer. In its current development it is a limited tool, but it has a very bright future. Spontaneous remissions of cancer and other illnesses are thought to be related to a strengthening of the immune system.

The technique of immunotherapy has a long-standing history. Its first use was as Coley's toxin in the 1880s to control bacterial infections. It was not known at the time how these toxins worked, but over the years more information has gradually accumulated. The Coast Guard can identify foreign or enemy ships just by looking at its flag; similarly, the immune system can differentiate the healthy cells of the body from the cancerous cells through flags of "self" and "non-self." Many tumor cells have special proteins on the cell surface called antigens which makes them look different to the eyes of the immune system. The immune system, in turn, makes a counter-attack force of special proteins called antibodies. This system, called "immune surveillance," can control cancer in the early stages, and was the basis for modern immunotherapy.

Vigorous attempts were made in the early 20th Century to stimulate the immune system. The first successes came in the treatment of melanoma and leukemias. Many patients with melanoma, up to 15 percent in some studies, were seen to have a spontaneous regression, not only of the primary tumor, but also of the metastases. The regression of melanoma or abnormal moles is from decreased pigment cells in those areas; when seen clinically, the areas look paler because the deep blue cancer cells were destroyed by the immune system. In some cases the primary melanoma disappeared, but the metastases remained. Patients with spontaneous remissions may have circulating anti-melanoma antibodies. This, too, shows the importance of the immune system in controlling cancer. A vaccine for melanoma is presently being tested at the M.D. Anderson Hospital in Houston, Texas.

The phenomena of spontaneous remissions is very exciting, and has also been seen in other cancers, such as cancer of the kidney, lymphatic cancers, and brain tumors. These remissions are not very well understood, but may be related to a strengthening of the immune system from a variety of causes. Cases have been reported of unexplained remissions linked to changes in diet, alternative therapies and to development of a positive attitude—to name a few. Perhaps they are due to some sort of natural miracle, as mentioned in the section on Lourdes that follows.

An important stimulant of the immune system against tuberculosis is the BCG vaccine, developed by researchers Calmette and Guerin. BCG has been found to be effective in a number of cancers, especially in the treatment of melanoma when injected locally into the lesions, and has been found somewhat successful in general stimulation of the whole immune system. Dr. Harry W. Herr of Sloan Kettering Memorial Institute feels that BCG vaccine instilled into the bladder regresses the bladder cancer.

Interferon was first discovered in 1957 and now has become commercially available for viral infections and cancers caused by viruses. Interferon works by interfering with the multiplication of the viruses. External genital warts in both men and women, which cause genital cancer, seem to regress with injections of interferon, as do laryngeal papillomas in children. Currently, more purified preparations are available with fewer side effects. Alpha interferon is being used to treat hairy cell leukemia and is successful in 95 percent of cases. Pentostatin is another agent and is used for the same purpose as interferon. It appears to be close to Alpha interferon in efficacy. Other cancers that respond to Alpha (α) interferon are chronic myelogenous leukemia, effective in 15-20 percent cases; Kaposi's sarcoma, effective in one-third of cases; helps 50 percent of patients with lymphomas; and 20-30 percent of cases with multiple myeloma.[53]

Interleukin II normally is produced by the immune system for fighting cancer and has been found to be helpful in treatment of a number of cancers. It is one of the biologic response modifiers and can stimulate killer cells (LAK cells). Interleukin-II treatment programs have been established by the National Cancer Institute in 14 of the 37 cancer centers in the United States, and programs are pending at ten more institutions. Start-up grants of between 80,000 and 100,000 dollars have been given to each center for LAK production. The National Cancer Institute has budgeted 2.5 million dollars to do research on Interleukin II, helped by a donation by Dr. Armand Hammer of 150,000 dollars for the research.[54] Now Interleukin II is being tried with AZT on AIDS patients.[55]

Other agents that are being used in immunotherapy treatments are monoclonal antibodies and colony stimulating factors. Monoclonal Antibody technology is a new approach that won a Nobel Prize for medicine in 1984 for G. Kohler and C. Milstein. Monoclonal (mono=one, clone=to copy) antibodies are of one specific type, and will go after whatever they have been designed to attack.[56]

IMREG-1 is one of the newer immunomodulators on the market and appears to slow down the disease progression in AIDS Related Complex (ARC). The president of IMERG-1, A. Arthur Gottleib, claims that this agent may be as good as AZT in helping to boost the immune system of AIDS patients.

Naltrexone (Trexan-Dupont) appears to boost the levels of endorphins, which apparently improves the communication between the brain and the immune system says Dr. Bernard Bihari. Bihari reported that 38 AIDS patients receiving the drug showed marked improvement in immune functions and survival rates.[57]

Met-encephalon is a drug that was used on 16 ARC patients; they showed improvements in weight gain, immune system functioning, T-cells and mood. None developed AIDS.[58]

Several other new drugs, like Thymosine injections and Levamisol, have also been found to stimulate the immune system.

Cancer Vaccinations

Marek's Disease in chickens and feline leukemia are diseases well known to us. They are now prevented by the vaccines available for cats and chickens. A similar approach has been successful for many viral diseases in humans, such as polio, smallpox and hepatitis B. However, there is a real need for vaccines against human papilloma virus and HTLV-1—which can cause lymphomas and leukemias, HIV, and Epstein-Barr Virus—to prevent many cancers by boosting the immune system against these deadly viruses. Vaccine research is currently being done with primates.

The Miracle of Lourdes

Throughout history there have been accounts of unexplained healings of diseases and injuries, accomplished by contact with the water or dirt of holy places, or of being touched by a holy person — miracle cures. Some of these have occurred in Lourdes, a small village located in southwest France that was practically unknown to the rest of the world until 1858. A 14-year-old girl named Bernadette claimed that the Blessed Virgin Mary appeared to her 18 times between February 11 and July 16, 1858. Only Bernadette seemed to have the visions. She was instructed by the Virgin Mary to dig at the ground and to wash and drink in the water of the spring. As she scratched at the dirt with her bare hands, water arose from the hole she had created. She was also instructed that a chapel was to be built on this miraculous site.

The water from this spring flows at the rate of 32,000 gallons a day. Nearly two million people visit the holy shrine every year for prayers and blessings, and to bathe in the holy water for healing.

A commission was appointed to study the claims of miraculous healings that took place at the Shrine at Lourdes. They reported by the year 1959 that out of the 5,000 reported cures 58 could be declared "miraculous."[59]

For further information about Lourdes, I recommend reading *The Miracle of Lourdes* by Ruth Cranston.[60]

LIVING WITH CANCER; TACTICS FOR SURVIVAL

Bonita Goldsmith died at age 52 of a cancer that had metastasized throughout her body in 1987. To outsiders, it seemed that her life had been snuffed out before its time. But her husband, family, and closest friends knew that she had been living with the diagnosis of cancer for 20 years. After having a radical mastectomy at age 32, a bout with lung cancer that was successfully treated with surgery and chemotherapy ten years after that, she suffered a final siege of illness that lasted for five years when the cancer spread to her hip socket and spine.

Why write about cancer survival in a book about cancer prevention? The premise here is to show that there are things that an individual can do to intervene or to make a difference even after they have developed the disease. In the earliest stages of initiation or promotion these interventions are of a precautionary or preventive nature. In the event of a diagnosable cancer, there is still a great deal that individuals can do to make a difference—and much of this has to do with emotional and mental attitude.

Dr. Mel Goldsmith recalls life of 20 years ago as busy and productive. He was putting his energies into building a psychiatric practice and taking up psychoanalytic training. His wife, Bonita, was raising three children, the youngest just six months old. The family had just moved into a luxurious home built on an old apple orchard in a southeastern Michigan suburb. It was a rustic spot, except that Dr. Goldsmith remembers that the apple orchard was sprayed frequently with pesticides. Within one year of the move, Bonita was diagnosed with breast cancer. She was one of five people on the block, all bordering that rustic apple orchard, who developed cancer.

"Bonita had two previous surgeries on that breast before the mastectomy, the first at age 22, which had both turned out to be benign papillomas," says Dr. Goldsmith. "When we first found out that the tumor was malignant, there was an impulse to think, 'Why me?', but we both knew that was a cop out," he says. "My wife was so young to have this disease, and we realized that her doctors were even more frightened than we were. We could not always rely on them for emotional support. The exams every three months after her mastectomy were particularly stressful. We concentrated on putting our energies into what was here and now, setting little goals for ourselves, six months or a year at a time."

For Dr. Goldsmith and his wife another important issue in living with, and rising above, the stress of a cancer diagnosis was openness to emotions. "My wife had no difficulty expressing what she felt, and that quality keeps one's eye on where one is, not where one was or wants to be.

"Fortunately, we were able to share a profound attitude. We could think very deeply about the illness, but not brood over it. We laughed about it, and made fun of ourselves and the condition. Sure, there were crises, and I wouldn't always tell her all of my fears or cite statistics. Instead we would focus on what we could do, and there was always something we could do, always something that would work for a while. Bonita was a great reader, and as a housewife, she was interested in diet and nutrition. She was always reading, researching, and thinking about the things she could do to build up her immune system. When Norman Cousins' book *Anatomy of an Illness* was published, she was deeply touched by it. His attitude toward her illness was her attitude. Though she didn't conceptualize it, what he was doing made sense to her.

"We would reassure each other. Usually she would start by coming to me with her worries. We'd talk, and I would get her on track—at least that was how it looked to others. Really, she was the one who inspired me, because she had the extraordinary ability of detaching herself from what she was most afraid of. Bonita could laugh ten minutes after confronting the most anguishing problems, not out of denial, but just because she could think about the moment at hand. In many respects, the last five years were the best quality time that we had in our 32 year marriage. She needed chemotherapy once a week, and, as a physician, I could administer the shots. I would give them to her in the evening so she could go to sleep afterwards and avoid the worst effects of nausea. It became our disease, we shared it, and we lived those 20 years in a very personal way. I learned a great deal from her and from the way she lived her life."

Another book recommended to those persons suffering from cancer is called *Living with Cancer: Portraits of Twelve Inspiring People*, by Robert L. Shook.[61]

CHAPTER EIGHT NOTES

1. Richard Getty, and R. Good, "Occurrence of Malignancy in Immunodeficiency Diseases," *Cancer*, (July 1971)

2. M.F. Essex, *American Journal of Epidemiology*, Vol. 4, (1982)

3. Samuel Broder, *New England Journal of Medicine*, (Jan. 28, 1988)

4. David Baltimore, and Mark Feinberg, Whitehead Institute, *New England Journal of Medicine*, (Dec. 14, 1989)

5. J. Mann, and J. Chin, *New England Journal of Medicine*, (Aug. 4, 1988)

6. Donald P. Francis, CDC. *Primary Care & Cancer,* (May 1990)

7. *Primary Care and Cancer,* (May 1990)

8. Judy M. Ismach,"Hepatitis B Virus Infections," *Medical World News*, (Sept. 24, 1984)

9. FDA, "Hepatitis B," *Drug Bulletin*, (Nov. 1986)

10. David Shafritz, et.al., "Integration of Hepatitis B Virus DNA into Genome of Liver Cells in Chronic Liver Disease and Hepatocellular Carcinoma," *New England Journal of Medicine*, (Oct. 29, 1981)

11. *American Journal of Epidemiology*. Vol. 20, #4, (1984)

12. FDA, *Drug Bulletin*, (Aug. 1985)

13. "FDA Approval Sought for Alpha Interferon Treatment of Genital Warts," *New Medical Science*, (March 1986)

14. R. Richart, and K. Trofatter, *Medical Tribune*, (June 30, 1988)

15. Albert Singer, et.al., *British Journal of Medicine*, (August, 1985)

16. John Paul Micha, and Paul D. Silva, "Condyloma Acuminata and Related HPV Infections," *The Female Patient*, Vol. 11 (Aug. 1986)

17. I. Martinez, *Cancer*, (1969)

18. M.J. Champion, *The Lancet*. 1: (1985)

19. R. Barrasso, et.al., *New England Journal of Medicine*, (Oct.8, 1987)

20. Leslie Roberts, "Sex and Cancer," *Science*, (1986)

21. Ronald Moy, *Journal of the American Medical Association*, (May 12, 1989)

22. Mortimer J. Lacher, *Ca-A Cancer Journal for Clinicians*, (Nov. 1981)

23. Nicholas J. Vianna, et.al., "Extended Epidemics of Hodgkin's Disease in High School Students," *The Lancet*, (June 12, 1971)

24. Epstein, M.A., *The Lancet*, (1986)

25. Anupam Routh, et.al. *Archives of Dermatology*, (April, 1985)

26. Fontaine, R. E. and Istre, G. R., *Journal of the American Medical Association*, (Dec. 14, 1984)

27. John D. Vieta, and Guillermo Delgado, *Diseases of Colon and Rectum*, (Jan. 1976)

28. B. Calkins, and A. Mendeloff, *Epidemiological Reviews*. Vol. 8, (1986)

29. Lanza, Robert P., et.al., "Malignant Neoplasm Occurring After Heart Transplantation," *Journal of the American Medical Association*, (April 1, 1983)

30. Arlene Kantor, et.al. *American Journal of Epidemiology*, Vol. 126, #3 (1986)

31. Roberts, *Lancet,* (Oct. 9, 1976)

32. Volker Schneider, *Acta Cytologica*, (May, 1983)

33. Kay, *New England Journal of Medicine*, (May 5, 1983)

34. Peggy Mann, *Marijuana Alert*, (NY: McGraw-Hill, 1985)

35. Lourdes Corman, *Medical Clinics of North America*, (May 1985)

36. Ian D. Gardner, "The Relationship Between Aging and Susceptibility To Infection," *Geriatric Medicine*, Vol. 5, #3 (March 1986)

37. Barbara Schindler, "Stress Affective Disorder & Immune Function," *Medical Clinics of North America*, Vol. 69, #3, (May 1985)

38. National Cancer Institute and American Cancer Society, *Physician's Travel and Meeting Guide*, (Oct. 1989)

39. Vernon Riley, Pacific Northwest Research Fndtn., *Medical World News*, (Jan. 26, 1987)

40. Jemmott, et.al., *Science*, (Sept.83)

41. *Medical World News*, (Jan. 26, 1987)

42. Parkes, et.al., *British Medical Journal*, (1969)

43. Schindler, *Medical Clinics of NA*, (May, 1985)

44. William F. Ganong, *Hospital Practice*, (June 15, 1988)

45. Neil Graham, et. al., *American Journal of Epidemiology*, Vol. 124, #3. (1986)

46. "How Your Personality Affects Health," *Good Housekeeping*, (June 1983)

47. Corman, *Medical Clinics of NA*, (May 1985)

48. Kanofsky, et.al. *Medical Tribune*, (April 22, 1987)

49. Corman, L. *Medical Journal of North America*. July 1985

50. Univ. of California. *Prevention Magazine*, (March 1989)

51. Rick McGuire, "Running Immunity," *Medical Tribune*, (Nov. 24, 1988)

52. Susan Mulley, *Medical Tribune*, (May 3, 1990)

53. *Medical World News,* (July 25, 1988)

54. John Durant, Fox Chase Cancer Center in Philadelphia.

55. *Medical World News*, (July 25, 1988)

56. Council of Scientific Affairs, *Journal of the American Medical Association*, (April 3, 1987)

57. Bihari, *Medical World News*, (Aug. 8, 1981)

58. *Medical World News*, (Aug. 8 1988)

59. *New Catholic Encyclopedia*, Vol. 8, Pg. 1031-32

60. Cranston, Ruth. *The Miracle of Lourdes*. Image Books/Doubleday, 1988

61. Robert L. Shook, *Living with Cancer: Portraits of Twelve Inspiring People,* (Harper and Row, 1983)

CHAPTER NINE

HEREDITARY AND FAMILIAL CANCERS

In the past most cancers were thought to be hereditary and a natural consequence of growing old. Yet a large body of research in the 20th century has shown that environment can play a major role in the development of cancer. According to Dr. Henry T. Lynch of Creighton University, it is now estimated that heredity is responsible for about five to seven percent of total cancers in human beings. When all hereditary factors are taken into consideration, the figure could be up to 20-25 percent of all cancers.[1]

Studies of cancer patients have shown that up to ten percent have three or more relatives with cancer. If a parent, aunt, uncle or child has had cancer, it puts you at an higher than average risk. The role of heredity in cancer causation is not yet fully understood, but because of genetic research, is becoming more clear. From a preventive point of view, it is extremely important that certain individuals—those with a strong family history of cancer or precancerous conditions—be identified at an early age for cancer detection and also for counseling.

Hereditary cancer has three important characteristics. First, it affects family members early. For example, breast cancer occurs at around age 60 for the general population, but hereditary breast cancer strikes at about age 44. Second, within a family, a cancer may occur at multiple sites, or multiple types of cancers may be diagnosed. Third, other members of the family may also be affected by similar causes.

Two surveys were done on cancer patients in the same oncology clinic. In one, six percent of the patients with cancer had two or more relatives with cancer, and in the other, only 1.5 percent had relatives with cancer. In another clinic, 200 patients claimed that they had an immediate relative (a brother, a sister, or parents) with cancer.[2]

As discussed in the explanation on cells in chapter two on biology, changing a normal cell into a cancer cell involves two hits. The first hit initiates the cell and causes permanent damage or "mutation" to the genetic material of the cell by means of chemicals, viruses and radiation. This first hit or mutation primes the cell. The second hit is promotion and is absolutely necessary for an initiated cell to be changed into a cancer cell. The agents that bring about the first hit are called initiators, and those which bring about the second hit are called promoters. Before a normal cell will change into a cancer cell, both hits have to occur in sequence. Initiation is quick, while promotion is a prolonged process.

With hereditary cancers, these two hits can combine in several different patterns. Both hits can be either hereditary or environmental, or the first hit can be hereditary and the second environmental.

The true hereditary cancer is seen when a gene or number of genes have been inherited which predispose the offspring to higher incidence of cancers. These genes can be in a "dominant pattern" where at least half of the offspring will get that cancer, or in a "recessive pattern," causing a small percentage to develop cancer. When a particular defective gene or genes that predispose an individual to a particular cancer cannot be identified, but a family develops certain cancers consistently at a high rate, it is called "familial cancer."

Some cancers may appear to be hereditary, but are actually environmental. For example, although exposure of a pregnant woman to smoking or alcohol may cause development of childhood cancers, this is not truly "hereditary cancer." Similarly, some cancers are seen in clusters; these are a result of family's or a community's common exposure to an environmental cancer-causing agent. "Cancer clusters" also are not considered hereditary.

DOMINANT INHERITANCE

In dominant inheritance, definite genes have been identified. Approximately 200 different genetic disorders are associated with higher risk for cancer. Here, at least half of the offspring may develop cancer and several generations may be affected. Three common examples of dominant inheritance are retinoblastoma, an eye tumor found in children, polyps in the colon, or Wilm's tumor, a kidney cancer in children.

RECESSIVE INHERITANCE

In these kinds of cancers, the first hit comes from heredity and the second from the environment. Weak or fragile chromosomes that lack the ability to repair genetic materials are attacked. An example of a recessive inheritance is a skin condition called Xeroderma Pigmentosa. Patients with this condition are instructed not to go out into the sun; their skin is not able to repair the damage to the genetic material by sunlight and they will develop skin cancers.

Another example is a condition called Ataxia telangiectasia. Patients with this condition have an immune deficiency and are at a 61-184 times higher risk for developing cancer—particularly lymphomas, leukemias, breast cancer and many others.[3] In a condition known as Fanconi's anemia, the liver is very sensitive to steroid medications; if anemic patients are treated with steroids, they may develop liver cancer. This condition affects one in 120,000 births and is almost always fatal by age 20.[4]

Other hereditary conditions can put people at higher risk for cancer. For example, twins or patients with Down's Syndrome are at a higher risk for leukemia. Similarly, patients with dysplastic, or abnormal, moles are at high risk for malignant melanoma. Also, patients with the hereditary condition of neurofibromatosis, made famous by the "Elephant Man," are at higher risk for many cancers such as brain tumors.

DEFECTIVE ENVIRONMENT DURING PREGNANCY

A defective environment during pregnancy is an example of a condition in which several children in the same family may be affected, but it is not considered a heredity cancer. We all know there may be poisons or medications the mother has been exposed to during pregnancy which will pass through the placenta and affect the fetus. The Thalidomide tragedy, where pregnant women took sleeping pills and their babies were born without arms and legs as a result, is an example. The drug DES has also caused birth defects and cancer in babies.

Smoking and drinking alcohol can cause many problems during pregnancy, both to the mother and to the fetus. Drinking alcohol may cause a form of mental retardation in fetuses. Called "fetal alcohol syndrome," these babies are at a three times higher risk for getting cancer. A similar syndrome, "fetal tobacco syndrome," has been described among women who habitually smoke during pregnancy. It can cause prematurity, low birth weight, and many childhood cancers such as leukemia and Wilm's tumor.

190

Even hormone levels in a mother's blood can affect the fetus. If the estrogen level is very high, the genitalia in the male fetus may not grow properly. These male babies are born with a condition called undescended testicle, which puts them at a 700 times higher risk of cancer of the testicles.

CANCER FAMILY SYNDROME

Hereditary cancers are usually inherited through a single gene, but in a "cancer family" multiple genes are inherited. The risk of developing cancer among different relatives in a cancer family can be up to 50 percent in first degree relatives.[5] There are two categories of cancer in these families. One is the Li-Fraumeni type, where varied types of cancers are seen in different relatives. The second is the Lynch type, where the same cancer affects many different relatives.

In the Li-Fraumeni type, which is named for Doctors Frederick Li and Joseph Fraumeni Jr., aggregate multiple cancers in the same families arise in different tissues at an early age, such as in soft tissue sarcoma, breast cancer and other cancers as well.

In the Lynch type, which is named after Dr. Henry T. Lynch, a prominent hereditary cancer researcher at Creighton University, two or more family generations are seen with cancers of the large bowel and uterus, usually diagnosed at an early age; and many patients have multiple primary tumors. Dr. Lynch's cancer research clinic focusses on counseling and early detection of hereditary cancer. Similar work on hereditary cancer is being done in other universities.

SECOND CANCERS IN A PAIRED ORGAN

Patients with hereditary cancers in a paired organ like breasts, testicles, ovaries, etc., are at higher risk for cancer in the second organ after cancer in the first one. For example, patients with cancer in one breast are at five to ten times a higher risk of developing a new cancer in the remaining breast.

HEREDITARY OR FAMILIAL CANCERS IN ADULTS

Breast Cancer

Research has shown that approximately ten percent of breast cancer patients have two or more close relatives with breast cancer.[6] However, a family history of breast cancer does not seem to put a woman at a high risk for breast cancer. Nevertheless, as this cancer is the number one killer of American women, it is important to analyze the risk factors.

There are three main considerations in hereditary breast cancer:[7]

1. Premenopausal or postmenopausal status of the affected woman,
2. Laterality, or whether the cancer affects one or both breasts,
3. Generation, or whether the breast cancer affects the family in sisters of the same generation, or in mothers and daughters.

The risk factors for breast cancer in the same generation are as follows: if two sisters are both premenopausal, an occurrence of breast cancer in one puts the other at a risk of 18 percent if only one breast is affected; the risk goes up to 50 percent if both breasts are affected. If the affected woman is postmenopausal, and the cancer affected only one breast, the risk to the sister is not higher than the average life-time risk of all women in the United States. This risk is ten percent.

In two generations the risks are much higher. If a mother has one affected breast at premenopausal age, the risk to the daughter is 33 percent; if both breasts are affected in the mother, risk to the daughter goes up to 50 percent. If the mother happens to be postmenopausal, the risks are much lower to the daughter.

If one generation is premenopausal and the second generation is postmenopausal, the risk to the daughter is 10 percent if the mother has cancer in one breast, and 23 percent if both breasts are affected. If both generations are postmenopausal, if the mother has cancer in one breast, the risk to her daughter is 16 percent, and if both breasts are affected, the risk goes up to 28 percent.

Put simply, a woman is at a higher risk for breast cancer if her mother or sister had a premenopausal breast cancer; the risk is greater if both breasts were affected.

If there is an extremely high rate of breast cancer in a woman's relatives, some surgeons will occasionally recommend a prophylactic mastectomy for her. However, the best way to handle the situation is to keep a close watch on persons at high risk, with breast self-examination, physician's exam and mammogram.

Colon Cancer

Colon cancer also appears to cluster in some families. There is a two to three times higher risk of colon cancer in the immediate relatives of patients with colorectal cancer.[8] This cancer often begins with benign polyps, but it can develop without polyps as an intermediate step. There are a number of related conditions affecting young patients that cause their colons to become covered with polyps, which, in turn, may become cancerous. These persons should have a close follow-up, with a physician checking the occult blood in the stool and performing a colonoscopy. These polyps should be removed surgically if they show evidence of developing into cancer. Surgical removal of the whole colon may be necessary if polyps arise simultaneously at multiple sites on the colon, but can be avoided if enough preventive steps are taken to monitor the polyps.

There is a special category of patients, termed Family Polyp Syndrome (FPS), where multiple generations in families are affected with polyps in the colon at a young age. Their chances of getting colon cancer can be nearly 100 percent. These patients need frequent contact and follow-up with their physician. A high fiber diet seems to help lower the risk for cancer of the colon in these patients.

Other hereditary conditions that may put persons at higher risk for colon cancer are Gardner Syndrome and Turcot Syndrome. Polyps can also arise in a non-familial fashion, which can raise the risk of cancer of the colon.

Ovarian Cancer

Incidence of ovarian cancer appears to be increasing, especially in Western countries. It follows an inheritance pattern similar to that of breast cancer. The immediate relatives of patients with cancer of the ovary are at three-and-a-half times the risk of developing the same, and relatives once removed are at three times the risk.[9]

The same chromosome abnormalities or similar derangements that have been found in patients with a hereditary type of ovarian cancer have been discovered in daughters and granddaughters. These have a 50 percent chance of developing the disease. There is now a blood test available for early detection of cancer of the ovary. If you are at high risk, Dr. Henry T. Lynch suggests prophylactic removal of both ovaries.

Testicular Cancer

Sometimes the estrogen hormone levels of pregnant women become abnormally high. This is often manifested in severe morning sickness. These excessively high hormonal levels can lead to an undescended testicle in the male fetus that may put the infants at higher risk for testicular cancer.[10] Undescended testicles are a common problem in young boys, and can be commonly diagnosed by the age of four months. Drs. Keith Schulze and Ronald Pfister of University of Colorado Health Science Center offer the following recommendations for follow-up: by age two these boys should be seen by a urologist; if testicles are still undescended by age 14, they should be surgically removed to prevent cancer. These young males who are at risk should

193

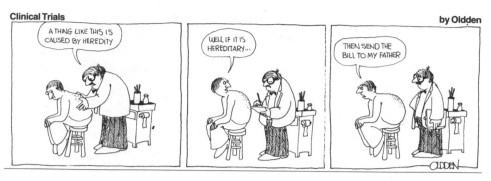

Reprinted with permission by *Medical Tribune* - Clinical Trials, May 13, 1987 p.19.

be taught testicular self-exam, and parents should also learn how to do a testicular examination on their babies.

Dysplastic Moles and Malignant Melanoma

Some people are at a higher risk of skin cancer because of their family history or an inherited skin type which may be highly sensitive to exposure to the sun. This phenomenon has been seen with one type of skin cancer in particular, called malignant melanoma. Malignant melanoma patients are often affected at a younger age, and multiple lesions are common.

Dysplastic nevi, which are abnormal moles, are another condition which may run in families. They are pre-cancerous and need careful follow-up. Patients with abnormal moles are also at very high risk for developing malignant melanoma during their lifetime. Families with many members having abnormal moles and with histories of melanoma should be classified as melanoma-prone. They are at the highest risk for developing melanoma, and the risk may increase to nearly 100 percent over their lifetime.

In an analysis done on 14 melanoma-prone families, the different members of these families with abnormal moles were identified and screened. Eight to twelve percent were found to be likely to have melanomas.

The risk of melanoma goes up to 50 percent in the immediate relatives of melanoma patients, given enough time. The lifetime risk of these relatives with abnormal moles may approach 100 percent. The conclusion of this analysis was that the members of melanoma-prone families with the highest risk are the ones who have both abnormal moles and histories of melanoma.[11]

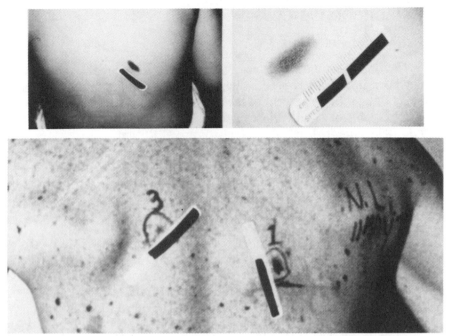

This patient with dysplastic nevus syndrome has had five separate primary melanomas. Several other family members have the syndrome. The mole in circle #3 and those on the left side of the lower part of the back are all dysplastic nevi. The lesion in circle #1 is an early superficial spreading melanoma. Note how much larger and more deeply pigmented it is compared with the preneoplastic moles.

Reprinted with permission from the Journal of the American Medical Association, Vol. 251, #14, April 13, 1984, ©1984, American Medical Association, and Kenneth A. Arndt, M.D.

Familial malignant melanomas constitute up to six percent of all malignant melanoma cases; the number goes up to 44 percent in those cases with multiple primary malignant melanomas. According to Dr. Alfred Kopf and associates of the New York University Melanoma Cooperative Group, familial melanomas are seen at a younger age at first diagnosis, and at multiple sites, usually in families from northern European and Celtic backgrounds.[12]

Since there is an eight to twelve times increase in incidence of melanoma in relatives of melanoma patients, Dr. William F. Duggleby and associates recommend a close surveillance of families of patients with a history of melanoma.[13]

CHILDHOOD CANCERS

Retinoblastoma

Retinoblastoma is a cancer of the eye, seen in one out of 15,000 newborn infants. It is predominantly seen in children younger than four years of age. Sixty percent of these cases are sporadic, occurring without a family history, and the remaining 40 percent can be classified as familial—inherited in a dominant pattern.[14] Recent genetic research has paved the way to predict which children are at risk for development of retinoblastoma. Until high-risk children reach the age of two-and-a-half, they should have regular eye exams by an ophthalmologist. Genetic counseling is very important to help families at high risk.

Wilm's Tumor

Wilm's tumor is a cancer of the kidney. In 20 percent of patients this appears to be familial, or inherited in a dominant pattern, and the rest are sporadic and appearing without a family history.

Brain Tumors

Neurofibromatosis was made famous by a patient, Joseph Merrick, more widely known as the "elephant man." It is seen in one in 3,000 live births, and nearly 80,000 Americans suffer from it. These patients are at high risk for many cancers, including leukemia and brain or nerve tumors.[15]

Fortunately, brain tumors are rarely seen in children. But, as with other childhood cancers, brain tumors are seen 20 times more frequently in relatives of brain tumor patients.

Neuroblastoma is the most common type of brain tumor in childhood and has been found to be familial in four out of five cases.

GENETIC COUNSELING

Genetic counseling is a new field in cancer prevention. Because ten percent of cancer patients have relatives with cancer, many cancer centers in the United States have opened new clinics in this field of preventive oncology. Therefore, such families at high risk are identified at an earlier age and can receive proper treatment. Occasionally, prophylactic treatment is advised, as in the case of patients with polyposis of the colon who are almost certain to develop cancer.

Early detection by periodic exam in high risk individuals is critical.

Genetic counseling facilities or referral to such facilities should be available through most cancer centers or hospitals. One of the units that specializes in the hereditary cancerous and hereditary precancerous diseases is the Hereditary Cancer Institute at Creighton University, Omaha, Nebraska 68178. Telephone: (402) 422-6237.

CHAPTER NINE NOTES

1. Arthur Holleb, *Cancer Book*. p.249, (New York: Doubleday, 1986)

2. John Mulvihill, "Cancer in Families," *New England Journal of Medicine,* (June 13, 1985)

3. Michael Swift, *New England Journal of Medicine,* (May 21, 1987)

4. *Medical Tribune,* (July 16, 1986)

5. Richard R. Love, and John F. Morrissey, *Archives of Internal Medicine,* (Nov. 1984)

6. Ruth Ottman, et al., "Familial Breast Cancer in Population — Based Series," *American Journal of Epidemiology,* Vol. 123, #1, (1986)

7. Patricia Kelly, and D.E. Anderson, *Post Mastectomy Reconstruction.*

8. Randall W. Burt, "Dominant Inheritance of Adenomatous Colonic Polyps and Colorectal Cancer," *New England Journal of Medicine,* (June 13, 1985)

9. Joellen Schildkraut, and W. Douglas Thompson, *American Journal of Epidemiology,* Vol. 128, #3

10. Andrew Moss, *American Journal of Epidemiology,* Vol 124, #1, (1986)

11. Mark H. Greene, National Cancer Institute, Second World Congress on Cancers of the Skin in New York, *Skin and Allergy News,* Vol. 16, #6

12. Alfred Kopf, et. al., "Familial Malignant Melanoma," *Journal of the American Medical Association,* (Oct. 1986)

13. Duggleby, et.al., *American Journal of Epidemiology,* Vol. 114, #1 (1981)

14. David Yandell, et.al., *New England Journal of Medicine,* (Dec. 21, 1989)

15. Vincent Riccardi, "Von Recklinghausen Neurofibromatosis," *New England Journal of Medicine,* (Dec. 31, 1981)

CHAPTER TEN

POLLUTION OF AIR, WATER AND FOOD

"Give a hoot—don't pollute." This catchy phrase was thought up by environmentalists in the early 70s and cropped up on bumper stickers. People began to take notice, marking a significant change of attitude and a deepening awareness of the tragic pollution of our environment. Concern for the environment has become more widespread, especially since such publicized disasters as the Exxon-Valdez oil-tanker accident in Alaska, spilling a vast quantity of oil into the sea.

The air we breathe, water we drink, food we eat, homes we live in and offices and factories where we work—have all become polluted. In the 1980s, pollution came not just from dirt or bacteria, but from the residue of more than 60,000 chemicals that "hang around" in our environment. We live in a "chemical soup," and our increased exposure to such pollutants can lead to an increase in many cancers.[1]

The earth we inherited was not pristine to begin with. Underground deposits of asbestos, radon gas and minerals like arsenic have contributed to "natural" pollution. However, human activities and technological progress have compounded the situation.

Extreme pollution cases of gigantic proportions usually make newspaper headlines: accidents such as the fire at the nuclear power plant in Chernobyl, U.S.S.R., the fire at the chemical manufacturing

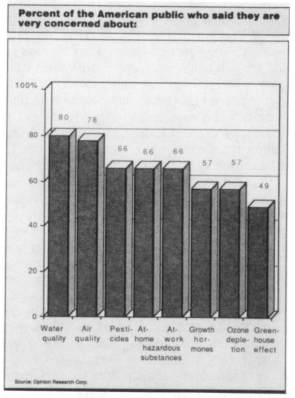

Percent of the American public who said they are very concerned about:

Source: Opinion Research Corp.

Reprinted with permission from Opinion Research Corporation, Aug. 1989.

plant in Bhopal, India, or even Three Mile Island in the United States, were well publicized. Less noticeable, but equally or more dangerous in terms of causing cancer, is what is known as chronic pollution. Chronic situations come about more gradually, after years of use and misuse.

All pollution is interconnected and, unfortunately, forms its own murky biological chain. For example, suppose you spray a pesticide on fruits and vegetables in your garden. (We'll use pesticide here, but any potentially carcinogenic material that can be airborne such as asbestos could also illustrate the same phenomenon.) Because the pesticide is an aerosol, it goes into the air which you inhale. Some lands on the fruits and vegetables, leaving a residue which remains on the food you eat, so you will ingest a small amount. Because these chemicals are so persistent, they do not dissolve; they linger in the soil until melting snow or rain water washes them off into the nearest river, which may be the source of your drinking water. The aquatic life in the river, especially fish, become contaminated. Smaller fish and insects can absorb these chemical pollutants. They, in turn, are eaten by larger fish, which are eaten by — ? You guessed it. The moral is: the things you use or throw away—don't always just go away. They become part of a continuous chain, and we will come into contact with them again. The supposition that air, water and soil have an unlimited capacity to absorb anything and everything that we choose to dump upon it is simply not true. And these pollutants will always come back to haunt us.

The exact percentage of cancers caused by pollution is not fully known because pollution is so widespread. Some authorities feel that the percentage could be extremely high, up to 20-40 percent. The pattern of cancers caused by pollution also varies. Pollution may cause an isolated case of cancer, affect the whole family, many people in the same neighborhood, or a wide geographic area—depending upon the distribution of the pollutants.

Cancer clusters are a polluted area in which a special pattern of cancers arises. Such "clusters" can be traced to exposure to a single cancer causing agent from an isolated source—similar to an hereditary or a familial type of cancer. For example, asbestos workers may carry asbestos home in their clothes, putting other members of the family at higher risk for cancer. Similarly, benzene workers bringing benzene residuals home in their clothing are exposing other people in the home to benzene and a higher risk of leukemia. Farm workers who are exposed to pesticides put themselves and their families at higher risk for cancer. A similar situation has been seen in people drinking polluted water from living near a toxic dump.

In general, research into these cancer clusters has been inconclusive. However, a cluster was seen in McFarland, California, a small town of 6,000, and described in the *Medical Tribune*.[2] Over the ten year period 1975-1985, there were eleven cases of childhood cancers—ten times the expected rate. The governor declared a state of emergency in the area. Dr. Jerome Marmorstein suspected that the culprit was the pesticide DBCP (2-dibromo, 3 chloropropane) contaminating the deep water wells in McFarland. Now all townspeople are being screened for contamination with the pesticide.

Dogs may react to cancer causing chemicals similarly to human beings, according to a study done by prominent authorities from the National Cancer Institute. In the 8,760 dogs they studied in 13 veterinary clinics, they found that the higher rates of bladder cancers in dogs in certain areas corresponded well with higher rates of industrial activity in the area. In dogs, cancer shows up in ten years, half the time it takes in a human being. If your pet dog has bladder cancer, it is possible you could be living in an area of industrial pollution.[3]

WATER, WATER EVERYWHERE AND NOT A DROP TO DRINK?

The quality of water has been an important concern throughout recorded time. Even in ancient societies that had no access to scientific proof, the beneficial properties of wholesome water was recognized.

The cholera epidemics which devastated English communities throughout the 1800s gave the earliest signs that water could transport infectious bacterial disease. During this time, Dr. John Snow, a London physician, knew that water was somehow responsible for the epidemic, but didn't know why or how. He broke the handle of the water pump that was the water source for a highly infected area, and the epidemic ceased dramatically. This was in 1854, about 50 years before scientist Louis Pasteur established the "germ" theory of disease.

Many worrisome waterborne diseases such as typhoid and cholera were prevalent in the United States at the turn of the 20th century. New methods of water purification were devised and legislated into effect throughout the country, and, as a result, typhoid was wiped out as an epidemic disease.

Water has become vulnerable to many new infiltrators with the advent of the petrochemical era. There are more than 700 organic chemical contaminants found in drinking water supplied by our nation's public water systems.[4] This figure probably represents only a "tip of the iceberg." Within the next few years it is proposed that 83 of the total number of the contaminants will be regulated; 40 of these are known carcinogens.

The common pollutants of water are inorganic, organic and radiation particles. Among the inorganic contaminants, arsenic, lead and nitrates are the most commonly seen. Organic pollutants are mostly pesticides, and radiation comes from underground radium. The type of contamination depends upon the source of water supplies-surface or ground water.

Water Supply Sources

Water supplies for human consumption come from two sources: surface water from rivers, ponds, reservoirs, and lakes; and ground water from shallow and deep wells. Surface water and shallow wells are subject to the same sources of contamination from human activity. The pollutants that leak into surface water come from direct industrial discharges, leaky landfills, illegal dumping by individuals and industry, and leaking underground storage tanks. Deep wells tend to get contaminated from natural sources of pollution such as underground radioactivity, asbestos deposits, arsenic and the like.

Surface waters and shallow wells are commonly contaminated by heavy metals, tar compounds, petrochemicals like benzene, dyes, pesticides, gaseous residues from plastic and rubber, asbestos fibers, PCB, PBB, and dioxin. All these are among 350 common carcinogenic contaminants that have been found in surface water in the five Great Lakes, our nation's largest inland body of water. At one time, it was thought these chemicals were safely buried at the bottom of the lakes after they were dumped. We now realize that their natural longevity, in combination with wave action after winter storms, stirs these chemicals up from the bottom and gives them another life.[5] As a result, the fish in the Great Lakes are developing cancerous tumors and birth defects. Lake trout cannot reproduce because the water is too toxic. The gulls, terns and cormorant in Green Bay, Wisconsin, suffer from a lethal beak deformity called crossed-beak.[6] One of the main rivers that feeds the Great Lakes is the Rouge River, very close to my home, and I can see for myself the murkiness of the water. It carries industrial discharges from the plants located along its banks and takes the pollutants to the Great Lakes. Congressman John Dingell feels the Rouge River is the largest single point source of pollution to the Great Lakes.[7]

Similarly, other lakes and rivers are becoming polluted. They have become the dumping ground for toxic chemicals, according to a report released by the National Wildlife Federation.[8] The fish in them are tainted with the pollutants, and are developing cancer at alarming rates. For example, 80 percent of two year old brown bullheads from the Black River near Cleveland and almost 100 percent of the Atlantic teem from the Hudson river near New York City have cancerous tumors.[9] John Black, a cancer researcher of Rosewell Park Memorial Institute in Buffalo, warns against eating tainted fish; he compares the risk of eating fish containing five PPM (parts per million) of suspected carcinogens to drinking Great Lakes water for 1,000 years.[10]

If possible, one should eat fish caught in the open sea; pregnant women and lactating mothers should be especially wary of fish taken from polluted waters.

The first research study to determine a link between cancer incidence and quality of water was carried out in the 1970s. The subject of the study was that all-American waterway, the Mississippi River. In 1974, the Environmental Defense Fund released a draft report that there were high rates of cancer deaths among people living near the Mississippi who used this as their principal water source. Drinking water for the City of New Orleans, located at the mouth of the Mississippi, was notorious, containing over 200 chemical pollutants. The river literally has been a drain pipe for half of the United States.

A study between 1960 and 1975 by Dr. Marise Gottlieb and colleagues of Tulane University School of Medicine in New Orleans studied 13 Mississippi River parishes in Louisiana utilizing cases of 17 cancer sites, primarily of the gastrointestinal (rectum) and genitourinary (bladder) tracts. The study found significant excess risk for cancer in the populations who drank Mississippi water (rectal cancer in males, and breast cancer in females) compared with those who drank surface waters and pre-chlorinated water supplies typical of larger communities.[11] Fortunately, more recent reports indicate that Mississippi river water is becoming cleaner.

Studies in Iowa done by Dr. Peter Isacson compared surface to ground water and found that industrial pollutants such as the volatile organic compounds such as dichloroethane (a solvent) were related to cancers of the colon and rectum, and the metal nickel to cancers of the bladder and lung. He also found that deeply imbedded ground wells often contained contamination from underground radiation or asbestos supplies and were tied with higher incidence of cancers like leukemia and gastrointestinal cancers.[12]

Another example of surface water contamination is in the Chesapeake Bay, once the nation's most fertile fishing ground. The delicate balance of the ecosystem has been tipped due to industrial discharges, sewage treatment plant discharges, and pesticide and fertilizer run-offs in the surrounding area.

What are other sources of danger to our water supplies? One is illegal dumping by industry. Such action caused the toxic pollution at Love Canal in New Jersey, where the soil and water became so polluted that an entire community had to be evacuated.

Another source comes from leaks in underground storage tanks (L.U.S.T.) which contain gasoline and dry cleaning agents. There are 4.8 billion gallons of gas which contain lead and benzene stored in underground tanks throughout the United States. Rusting tanks often spill these contents into the ground soil and water.[13]

The examples above are of pollution in surface waters, but deep well water also gets polluted at the source. There have been a number of studies of deep well water in a number of countries. For example:

• The water in Taiwan—high in arsenic—has been shown to be related to increased rates of skin cancer in the Taiwanese.

203

- Water in some Canadian provinces like Quebec have high levels of asbestos fiber, and asbestos is held in high suspicion of causing gastrointestinal cancers in Canadian cities like Toronto, Ottawa and Montreal, with high incidence of gastrointestinal and lung cancers.[14]
- Areas of phosphate mining in South Florida were found to correspond with increased levels of radioactivity in the ground water (>5SpCi/L), inducing higher rates of leukemia as compared to areas with low radioactivity levels.[15]

Transporting Water

Water not only gets contaminated at the source but also in transport. Water often runs through asbestos cement pipes or pipes in homes which are sometimes soldered with lead, corroding over time. These pipes may release carcinogenic contaminants like asbestos, cadmium and lead into our water. Plastic pipes may leach vinyl chloride and many other contaminants, and pollutants from the neighborhood can leach through the plastic into the water.

Water Purification by Chlorination

It was well known by the early 1970s that while chlorine reduced bacteria in water, it reacted with the organic substances in water to form chloroform and related compounds known as chlorinated methanes or Trihalomethanes (THM). These carcinogenic chemicals were therefore in many finished public drinking and water supplies treated with chlorine. Chloroform has even been found in water in the hottest showers.[16] Several cancers such as bladder, brain, non-Hodgkin's Lymphoma and kidney, have been correlated with THM levels. THM has the strongest association with bladder cancer.[17] A study by Dr. Charles Lawrence found a high rate of colorectal cancer in New York among white male teachers exposed to THM (chloroform) in drinking water, as compared to the general population.[18]

Public drinking water often has fluoride added to it for its beneficial effects in dental cavity prevention. However, fluoride in the water is now being linked to bone cancer, according to a recent study done by the National Toxicology Program.[19]

What Can We Do To Improve the Quality of Water?

The key for us is to *prevent* pollution of water in the first place. This can be facilitated by using minimal amounts of hazardous products and disposing of them in ways that are not intrusive to the water and soil around us. For example, it is better to dispose of residual amounts of paint thinner as a hazardous waste in a closed container, rather than throwing it into the backyard soil or down the drain.

If your water does not taste good or does not look clean, and you know of toxic dumps or industrial activity in your immediate area, you can have it tested several ways:

- Call the local health department.
- Have it tested at an Environmental Protection Agency certified laboratory.
- Buy water treatment equipment. Be sure the salesman is reputable, the equipment has a Gold Seal validation by the WQA (Water Quality Association), and that it has a warranty. The equipment must be installed and maintained.

If you have questions about your water, you can write to:

Water Quality Association   EcoWater Systems, Inc.
P.O. Box 606   P.O. Box 64420
Lisle, Il 60532   St. Paul, MN 55164 (800) 545-1780

One of the most important steps to maintaining water quality is to make sure it is not polluted at the source. As a good citizen, it is your duty to dispose of hazardous waste properly. Americans produce 148 million tons of municipal garbage yearly; yet only 15 million tons are recycled.[20] The best way to handle garbage at the present time is to do as much recycling as possible.

How to Dispose of Your Household Garbage

Garbage is more than just a nuisance. Many items that are frequently used around the house contain hazardous and toxic chemicals, so if they are disposed of with the general household garbage, they will pollute the landfill, the soil and water supply. Ultimately these toxins will end up in our food chain. Whether the cans and containers are full or empty, care should be taken to separate these toxic products from the routine methods of disposal. Some of the frequently used household items that are toxic are: pesticides and weed killers, pet and flea collars, no-pest strips, wood preservatives and stains, paints and varnishes, old art supplies, pool chemicals, chemicals used in photography, aerosol cans, used motor oil, lawn mower gasoline, engine de-greaser, battery fluid, car waxes and antifreeze fluid.

One way to handle disposal of these substances is to exchange them through community projects. As they say, "one man's garbage is another man's gold." Special days can be set aside for collections arranged through churches or community organizations.

Recycling and exchange are part of a new philosophy in waste management, integrated waste management. In this system the waste is separated into categories, some of it in landfills, some incinerated, some composted and recycled.[21]

AIR POLLUTION

Americans have spent 200 billion dollars on improving air quality over the past decade, according to a *Newsweek* report.[22] Again, this is not a new issue. Brick kilns used in the 12th century in England were observed to be spewing forth all sorts of contaminants into the air. The advent of the industrial revolution brought coal and petrochemicals into everyday use. Because of international political considerations, the nuclear industry has also expanded enormously as an alternative source of power to petrochemicals.

Acute situations of air pollution have been discussed. Equally serious is the ongoing situation, endangering to all of us. We have created all of the industries, automobiles and airplanes that put out hazardous air pollutants (HAPs) or "air toxins."

In general, air is more polluted in urban areas than in rural ones. Comparison of lung cancer rates among non-smokers in urban versus rural areas are two to three times higher.[23] Tobacco smoke and air pollution appear to act synergistically in producing cancer. The risk of lung cancer was four times higher in smokers exposed to air pollution compared to smokers without exposure to occupational air pollution says Dr. John Vena at the State University of New York in Buffalo.

The average American today spends 23 hours a day indoors. Nonetheless, the quality of outside air is very important, because indoor air quality depends upon it. If you are living in an area where there are a lot of industries, automobiles, or nuclear installations, naturally outdoor air is going to be more polluted and will pollute indoor air as well.

Outdoor air can be polluted by chemicals and nuclear materials. Chemicals come from many sources—both mobile and stationary. Mobile sources include: automobiles, planes and ships that release many carcinogenic materials in auto emissions.

There are two different types of air pollution. Our vehicles are responsible for one kind: they emit volatile gases mixed with fine particles that have been nicknamed "Los Angeles type" air pollution. The second type of pollution is created from stationary industries—mines and smelters—heavy on large particulates and dust, and is called the "London-type" of air pollution. The stationary sources include: fuel-combustion in coal fired plants, electrical generation and plants that convert coal into coke. Industrial sources include: asbestos-based industries, metallurgy operations, manufacture and use of petrochemicals and even gas stations. The solid waste disposal in landfills, toxic dumps, and incinerators, release a combination of air toxins. Forest fires are another source of pollution. They release many carcinogenic materials such as tar compounds.

People living near nuclear installations in general have been found to have higher than average rates of leukemias and brain tumors.

Indoor Air Pollution

We spend more and more time indoors, both for work and leisure. That makes air quality indoors very important for health and prevention of disease. This became even more important during the energy crunch of the 1970s when the national consciousness was raised to build more energy-efficient dwellings. Offices and homes were built with a special emphasis on being "air-tight" with a subsequent decrease in air exchange. The ventilation in homes is measured as air changes per hour (ACH). In normal homes, the ACH is about half to one-and-a-half, but in airtight houses, it can be one air change every five hours.[24] This air-tight feature was coupled with alternative home heating which released more pollutants with unexpected side effects. We started bottling up all of the filthy air contaminants such smoke, soot, germs, chemicals, radiation particles, and the list could go on and on.

Of course, inside air quality is dependent on outside air, but these indoor levels of contaminants can get two to five times higher than outside according to the EPA, dangerously high when air is not being exchanged frequently enough with outside air.[25] According to EPA's Lance Wallace, outdoor air pollution accounts for less then 25 percent of the nationwide exposure to air toxins—the homes are sickest of all buildings.

Indoor air can get polluted by soil and construction materials, human activity, and heating and cooking appliances. The dangers posed in construction from radon gas, asbestos, and formaldehyde have already been covered.

Smoking and Air Pollution

Among the many human activities that cause indoor air pollution, smoking is the number one cause. Smoking releases thousands of chemicals, enough to make a mini Love Canal of your home. Even though only 30 percent of American adults smoke, more than 50 percent of adults and 70 percent of children live in houses with at least one smoker.[26] (Rates of cancer due to second hand smoke is discussed in chapter three on tobacco.) In smoking households, not only are carcinogenic polycyclic hydrocarbons high, but benzene levels, which can cause leukemia in adults and children, increase too. Blood benzene levels in smokers are ten times higher compared to non-smokers, and benzene levels can be 50 times higher in homes with an adult smoker. Children living with smoking parents are at a higher risk for leukemia. Investigations on indoor air quality that were conducted by the National Institute for Occupational Safety (NIOSH) in 1983, found that smoking was a contributor in nearly every complaint. Improper ventilation was found to be the main problem in 48 percent of the investigated 203 complaints. NIOSH's recommendations from these investigations: intake of outside air must be four times higher when cigarette smoke is present in a building than when it is not.[27]

Other Activities

Hot showers, as mentioned already, can be responsible for production of chloroform in the houses with the levels four to five times higher than outside air when chlorine is added to the water.[28]

Clothes from the dry cleaning shop have solvents like TCE (trichloroethylene) and PCE (perchloroethylene). These should be aired out in the garage before they are taken inside the house—because the solvents remain in the clothes and can contaminate the air.

An aerosol spray can, no matter what its contents, may contain formaldehyde and methylene chloride. Cleaning fluids, pesticides, glues, paints and thinners, all add another dimension of pollution to the air we breathe. Air deodorizers and moth killing preparations contain a chemical which is a close cousin to benzene. It is called paradichlorobenzene and is a known carcinogen.

Cooking and Heating Appliances

The second major source of indoor air pollution comes from cooking and heating appliances. Many kinds of cooking and heating appliances can bring added pollution. For example, heating appliances are common causes of pollution in homes. Gas stoves give off the products of incomplete combustion containing carcinogenic materials. All gas appliances such as furnaces, gas water heaters and gas clothes dryers should be regularly inspected for malfunction or leakage. If the gas burner flame is yellow or orange instead of blue, it needs adjustment. Efficient exhaust fans are especially important. If there is no exhaust fan, a window should be left open. Gas stoves or ovens should not be used to heat your houses. You should *never* cook with charcoal inside the house.

Gas space heaters are another important source of pollution and need to be vented outside the room. Kerosene heaters, usually used in climates with milder winters, are more dangerous because they are not vented to the outside at all—the combustion products are released right into the room.

Fireplaces and wood burning stoves pollute both inside and outside air. Fireplace dampers should be open before lighting a fire and be kept open until the ashes have cooled down. In the United States there are more than 12 million wood burning stoves, and they contribute about 15 percent of the particulate emissions.[29] This kind of pollution is rampant in small towns. For example, half of the residents in the northern Michigan town of Mio own wood burning stoves. The town has so much pollution from the use of these stoves that driving through it in fall or winter was akin to driving through the smoke of a forest fire. The State of Michigan has recommended the use of catalytic converters, like those used on today's automobiles be used on these wood burning stoves.[30] The EPA is trying to establish regulatory standards, but the consumer should know that these stoves need to be carefully installed, with all exhaust pipes vented outside and checked periodically for leakage. Coal fired residential furnaces also have been found to release carcinogenic polycyclic hydrocarbons.[31]

Is Your House Getting Enough Fresh Air?

To maintain adequate quality of indoor air, you need an air change about every two hours. However, if there is a smoker in the house, you must increase the air change rate by at least four times.[32] If your house is too humid, or if your family experiences pollution related symptoms, your ventilation may not be adequate and needs to be increased. Radon kits have already been mentioned in chapter four.

Formaldehyde monitors manufactured by 3M and DuPont are available to homeowners. They are small plastic devices that can be hung in the house for a week and then sent back to be analyzed by the manufacturer.

Sick Building Syndrome

Beautiful skyscrapers of all colors and lights adorn most downtowns, but when you enter the building, you start sneezing or coughing. You discover that the skyscrapers may not be all that beautiful, because every time you walk into one, you begin to feel sick.

The "Sick Building Syndrome" is a modern disease caused by indoor air pollution. Office workers may feel sick, nauseated, or tired, with head and body aches when they are at work. These complaints were initially thought to be due to the poor attitude of the workers, but further investigation of these complaints showed that these symptoms were not psychological.

As more office towers are built, their central air systems consist of 15-20 percent of fresh air. The rest is recycled to save on heating and cooling costs. The result, of course, is that indoor air pollution levels rise. The pollutants found in office buildings come from many sources, such as plastic furniture, styrene, formaldehyde and benzene, solvents and glues, air sprays. smoke from cigarettes, and hydrocarbon and ozone exhaust from copiers.

The best solution is to open the windows and let the fresh air in.

MODERN FOOD — A CHEMICAL FEAST

Our food is derived from plant and animal sources, both of which are becoming increasingly polluted.

Animal, Bird and Fish Sources

The animals raised for slaughter, such as cattle and pigs, and birds such as chicken and turkeys, are raised on feed containing growth hormones. Therefore, DES and other residues can still end up on our dinner tables indirectly. Sometimes feed is contaminated with PBB. Wild animals and birds living in an area polluted with herbicides can also be contaminated.

Fish caught in polluted waters may be quite dangerous to eat because they can contain contaminants. Shell fish are the worst because of their ability, as a primitive form of fish, to store toxins. Fish caught from the Great Lakes show birth defects and cancerous tumors. A fisherman may not be aware if he's catching contaminated fish. The best thing to do is to clean the fish well and remove all the fatty portions, as shown in the diagram.

In summary, food not only gets contaminated at the source, but can be contaminated many places along the way. Storage of foods in silos using EDB, processing food with all kinds of additives to increase shelf life, curing food, cooking food by smoking, or storing food in plastic materials all may lead to further contamination.

Cleaning Great Lakes Fish

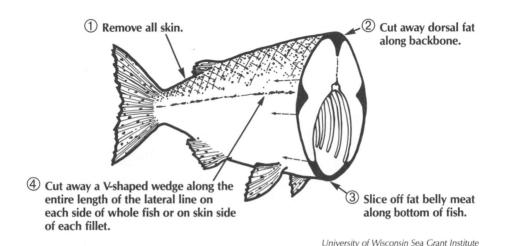

① Remove all skin.

② Cut away dorsal fat along backbone.

④ Cut away a V-shaped wedge along the entire length of the lateral line on each side of whole fish or on skin side of each fillet.

③ Slice off fat belly meat along bottom of fish.

University of Wisconsin Sea Grant Institute

Reprinted with permission from The University of Wisconsin Sea Grant Institute.

Plant Sources

Our convenient life style has led to widespread pollution of the environment, which is infiltrating the food chain. Plants, vegetables and fruits are grown with the assistance of soil-polluting chemicals like pesticides and fertilizers. The fertilizers contain nitrites and nitrates that contaminate the food and become nitrosamines in the stomach. High phosphate fertilizers contain radiation particles which have been found in tobacco leaves. Excessive use of pesticides can lead to residues on food. A recent example is the finding of the pesticide alar on peanuts and apples.

The air and water pollution will eventually end up in our soil and food. The routine Market Basket Surveys have shown pesticide residues on fruits, vegetables and grains and even the pesticide EDB (Ethylene Dibromide) in cookie mixes.

A landmark study done in Ontario, Canada, in 1986 by Kathleen Davis showed that people eat about eight times more toxic chemicals in food than they consume in the toxic chemicals in both air and water put together. Since *32* of these chemicals, including Dioxins and Dibenzo-furans (animal carcinogens) have been found in fresh meat, milk, vegetables and fruit grown in Ontario, it is suspected similar contamina-

211

tion is possible in the United States. One of the horrible side-effects of indiscriminate use of pesticides is the overgrowth of the fungus on grains and nuts which is giving rise to higher aflatoxin contamination of our food supply.

Fumigants like EDB are used to store the grain in silos and some amount does end up in commercially prepared mixes.

To avoid pesticide residues in food:

- Try to grow your own food as much as possible. Freeze or preserve it for winter months. You can also buy foods directly from small town local organic growers.
- Removing outer leafy portions of the vegetable can reduce pesticide residues. These outer portions contain most of the residues.

POLLUTION OF BREAST MILK

Breast milk is an outlet for the chemicals stored in the fatty tissues of the body. Whatever is stored in the fatty tissues will come out in the breast milk. A number of studies have shown that pesticides PBB and PCBs that are stored in a lactating woman's body have been detected in their milk. In a research report by Dr. Walter Rogan and his associates of the National Institute of Environmental Health Sciences, the recommendation was that lactating mothers should avoid eating fish caught from contaminated waters.[33] These women should also avoid excessive weight reduction during the time of breast feeding because that releases or mobilizes chemicals from the fat stores in the body.

According to experts in Michigan, women with PCB levels over ten parts per million in their breast milk should stop breast feeding because their infants are being overdosed on the toxic chemical.[34] Dr. Jeffrey Hergenrather and his associates from the Ethos Research Group and Dr. Eldon Savage of Colorado State University concluded that the breast milk of a vegetarian woman is the safest for infants because there is less chemical pollution.[35]

CHAPTER TEN NOTES

1. *American Journal of Epidemiology,* Vol. 124 #6, (1986)
2. *Medical Tribune,* (Jan. 14, 1988)
3. Howard Hayes, Jr., Robert Hoover and Robert Tarone, *American Journal of Epidemiology.* Vol. 114, #2, (1981)

4. Leonard Schuman, "Epidemiology of Environmental Carcinogens with Reference to Water Supplies," *Drinking Water and Human Health*, American Medical Association, Chicago, (1984)

5. *Detroit News*, (May 30, 1985)

6. Valdas V. Adamkus, "Toxic Pollutants and the Great Lakes," EPA, *Detroit News*, (July 1, 1986)

7. *Dearborn Press and Guide*, (Aug. 28, 1986)

8. National Wildlife Federation, *Air/Water Pollution Report*, (Aug. 14, 1989)

9. John Harshberger, *Environmental Digest/Science Digest*, 92/4:30, (April 1984)

10. John Black, *Doctor, I've Read...*, (April 1984)

11. Marise Gottlieb, et.al., *American Journal of Epidemiology*, Vol.116 #4 (1982)

12. Isacson, et.al., "Drinking Water and Cancer Incidence in Iowa," *American Journal of Epidemiology*. Vol. 121, #6 (1985)

13. R. Hawley Truax, "LUST in America," *Environmental Action*, (Sept. 1986)

14. Lincoln Polissar, et al., "Cancer Incidence in Relation to Asbestos in Drinking Water in the Puget Sound Region," *American Journal of Epidemiology*, Vol. 116, #2 (1982)

15. Gary Lyman, et.al., "Association of Leukemia with Radium Ground Water Contamination," *Journal of the American Medical Association*, (Aug. 2, 1985)

16. Isacson, *American Journal of Epidemiology*, (1985)

17. Kenneth Cantor, et.al., "Association of Cancer Mortality with Halomethanes in Drinking Water," *Journal of the National Cancer Institute*, 61:4 (Oct. 1978)

18. C. Lawrence, *Journal of the National Cancer Institute*, (March 1984)

19. National Toxicology Program, *Medical Tribune*, (Dec. 28, 1989)

20. Paul Rebis, *Health and Environmental Digest*, (Sept. 1987)

21. *Ibid.*

22. *Newsweek*, (Winter, 1985)

23. Bertram Carnow, *Environmental Health Perspectives*, Vol. 22, (1978)

24. Michael Lafavore, "Clean Air Indoors," *Rodale's New Shelter Magazine*, (1982)

25. *U.S. News and World Report*, p. 71-72 (Sept. 23, 1985)

26. Scott Weiss, "Indoor and Outdoor Air Pollution, and Airway Disease," *MediGuide to Pulmonary Medicine*, Vol. 3, #1

27. *Medical World News Report*, (Sept.9, 1985)

28. Rick McGuire, "Can't Hide from Pollution Indoors," *Medical Tribune*, (Jan. 7, 1987)

29. Lucy Johnson, "Pot Belly Smoke," *Environmental Action*, (Jan/Feb.1987)

30. *Detroit News*, (June 17, 1985)

31. G. Grimmer, Biochemical Institute of Environmental Carcinogens, Germany, *Cancer Letters*.

32. "Cigarette Smoke Involved in Most Indoor Air Pollutants," *Family Practice News*, (Aug. 1, 1985)

33. Walter Rogan; Anna Bagniewska and Terri Damstra, "Pollutants in Breast Milk," *New England Journal of Medicine*, (June 26, 1980)

34. *Medical World News*, (March 30, 1981)

35. Jeffrey Hergenrather, and Eldon Savage, et.al., *New England Journal of Medicine*, (March 26, 1981)

CHAPTER ELEVEN

EARLY DETECTION OF CANCER

SECONDARY PREVENTION

Secondary prevention is achieved by screening healthy individuals in high-risk populations for early detection and prevention of cancer. Screening can be done in a variety of ways, including the use of questionnaires to identify people at high risk of getting cancer, the creation of local and nationwide screening programs and cancer-related checkups.

The prevention of cancer has only been promoted by the medical community in the last 30 years, beginning with the American Cancer Society's recommendations for Pap smears. In the past, medical schools have often given less attention to prevention than to treatment of disease. Only recently have physicians been learning more about what measures may be valuable in the prevention of cancer.

It is important that physicians educate their patients about prevention during office visits, general exams and yearly checkups. Studies show that patients with a fatal cancer have a better chance at long-term survival if the cancer is caught at its earliest stages—before it spreads to more than one area of the body. Studies also say that patients who already have had cancer have a better chance of it recurring or that a second type of cancer will develop than the average person. These patients should be watched especially carefully.

How can we detect cancer early? There are three important ways:

I. By *assessing risk* and monitoring symptoms. You can begin to evaluate your own risk with questionnaires like the one given below. If physicians also watch for possible warning signs of cancer in their patients on a regular basis, there will be no delay in seeking the necessary medical care.

II. By learning the proper techniques of *self-examination*. Health education should be promoted so that people are given a chance to modify their lifestyles to lower their risk of developing cancer.

III. By undergoing periodic *physicals and lab tests* when indicated and having cancer related check-ups.

I. SELF-QUESTIONNAIRES TO ASSESS RISK

There are a variety of prescreening questionnaires that can be used to evaluate the risk for cancer.

Skin Cancer Questionnaire

A. Symptoms   YES NO

    1. Any history of skin cancer in the past? □ □
    2. Any rash or mole present for six months or more? □ □
    3. Any warts in the genital area? □ □
    4. Any colored moles with bluish, blackish or reddish tints? □ □
    5. Any itching or color changes in the moles? □ □

B. Risk Factors

    1. Do you have Blonde hair? Tan easily? Burn easily? □ □
    2. Family history of melanoma? □ □
    3. Any freckling on back? □ □
    4. Any Actinic Keratosis (sun-damaged skin areas) on skin? □ □
    5. More than three blistering sunburns in childhood? □ □
    6. Three or more outside summer jobs as a teenager? □ □

As the number of these risk factors increase, so does risk for melanoma. If you have three or more risk factors, you chances are 20-25 percent over a life time.

C. Health Habits   YES NO
1. Do you use sunscreens before going to the beach? ☐ ☐
2. Do you use sunlamps or tanning booths or beds? ☐ ☐

Breast Cancer Questionnaire

A. Symptoms   YES NO

1. Any history of a lump in the breast or
   enlarged glands in the arm pits? ☐ ☐
2. Any change in the skin of the breast, like dimpling? ☐ ☐
3. Any history of breast pain, other then during periods? ☐ ☐
4. Any change in the nipples? Rash or eczema? ☐ ☐
   Discharge from the nipple, watery or bloody? ☐ ☐
   Inverted nipple? ☐ ☐

B. Risk Factors

1. Family history of breast cancer in mother or sister
   less then 50 years of age? ☐ ☐
2. History of hormone use such as birth control pills, DES,
   or estrogens? ☐ ☐

C. Health Habits

1. Do you practice breast self-examination? ☐ ☐
2. When was your last mammogram? ☐ ☐
3. When was your last physical exam by a physician? ☐ ☐

Lymphatic Cancers and Aids Questionnaire

A. Symptoms   YES NO

1. Any enlarged lymph nodes in the neck, groin or armpits? ☐ ☐
2. Any fever without an obvious cause for a couple of weeks? ☐ ☐
3. Any severe weight loss (more then 20 pounds) within
   a couple of months? ☐ ☐
4. Continuous diarrhea for more than 3 weeks? ☐ ☐
5. Thrush in the mouth? ☐ ☐
6. Repeated infections like pneumonia? ☐ ☐

B. Risk Factors

A. Any history of homosexuality or multiple
   heterosexual partners? ☐ ☐
B. History of IV drug abuse? ☐ ☐
C. History of Blood Transfusion or Blood Products? ☐ ☐

Head and Neck Cancers

A. Symptoms   YES NO

    1. Any sores, white patches, or red patches in the mouth
       for more then a month?   ☐   ☐
    2. Any area of irritation in mouth caused by
       jagged tooth or dentures?   ☐   ☐
    3. Any difficulty swallowing or pain on swallowing?   ☐   ☐
    4. Any hoarseness or change in voice?   ☐   ☐
    5. Any obvious swelling in the front of the neck,
       sides or around the face?   ☐   ☐

B. Risk Factors

    1. Any history of chewing tobacco or smoking
       cigarettes, pipes, or marijuana?   ☐   ☐
    2. Alcohol use on daily basis?   ☐   ☐
    3. Any history of radiation to head and
       neck area in childhood?   ☐   ☐

C. Health Habits

    1. Do you practice mouth self-examination?   ☐   ☐

Female Genital Tract

A. Symptoms   YES NO

    1. Any history of unusual vaginal bleeding?   ☐   ☐
       In between periods?   ☐   ☐
       Six months after menopause or hysterectomy?   ☐   ☐
       After sex?   ☐   ☐
    2. Any genital warts on vulva or vagina or any enlarged
       lymph nodes in the groin?   ☐   ☐

B. Risk Factors

    1. Any history of hormone use?   ☐   ☐
       DES?   ☐   ☐
       Birth Control Pills?   ☐   ☐
       Post Menopausal Estrogens?   ☐   ☐
       Steroids?   ☐   ☐
    2. Any history of smoking?   ☐   ☐
    3. History of weight gain, 20 percent over
       the expected weight?   ☐   ☐
    4. Any history of operation on the cervix?   ☐   ☐

C. Health Habits   YES NO

   1. Any history of Pap smear?   ☐   ☐
     Colposcopy?   ☐   ☐
     D and C?   ☐   ☐

Kidney and Bladder Cancer

A. Symptoms   YES NO

   1. Any history of blood in the urine in the last six months? ☐   ☐
   2. Frequency and burning on urination?   ☐   ☐

B. Risk Factors

   1. History of tobacco use?   ☐   ☐
   2. Work in petrochemical industry?   ☐   ☐
   3. Exposure to dyes at home or in the work place? ☐   ☐
   4. Are you an avid fisherman using dyed earthworms? ☐   ☐

Lung Cancer

A. Symptoms   YES NO

   1. Any persistent cough or change in cough?   ☐   ☐
   2. Blood in the phlegm?   ☐   ☐
   3. History of repeated pneumonia?   ☐   ☐

B. Risk Factors

   1. History of smoking personally?   ☐   ☐
     Exposure to second-hand smoke?   ☐   ☐
   2. Work in asbestos factory or asbestos related work? ☐   ☐
   3. History of work in a foundry, rubber,
     plastic, petrochemicals?   ☐   ☐
   4. History of uranium mining or work with nuclear materials? ☐   ☐
   5. Any history of high radon levels at home?   ☐   ☐
   6. Family history of lung cancer?   ☐   ☐

C. Health Habits

   1. Do you eat a lot of fresh fruit and vegetables? ☐   ☐
   2. Do you take any vitamin supplements?   ☐   ☐
   3. When was the last chest x-ray?   ☐   ☐

Cancer of the Stomach

A. Symptoms   YES NO

   1. Any history of weight loss of more then 20 pounds
     in a couple of months?   ☐   ☐
   2. Persistent nausea or vomiting?   ☐   ☐
   3. Fullness after eating small meals?   ☐   ☐

Symptoms with Cancer of the Stomach *continued*

	YES	NO
4. Any history of ulcer?	☐	☐
5. Any history of anemia?	☐	☐
6. Any history of blood in vomit or tarry stools?	☐	☐

B. Risk Factors

	YES	NO
1. Do you smoke?	☐	☐
2. Do you eat a lot of cured, fermented or smoked foods?	☐	☐
3. Do you drink alcohol daily?	☐	☐

C. Health Habits

	YES	NO
1. Do you eat a well-balanced meal with fruits and vegetables?	☐	☐

Cancer of the Colon and Rectum

A. Symptoms

	YES	NO
1. Any history of bleeding from the rectum?	☐	☐
Fresh or tarry?	☐	☐
2. Any change in the bowel habits?	☐	☐
Constipation?	☐	☐
Diarrhea?	☐	☐
3. Any pain in abdomen or cramping at the time of bowel movement?	☐	☐
4. Any weight loss more then 20 pounds in a couple of months?	☐	☐

B. Risk Factors

	YES	NO
1. Do you eat a high fat, low fiber diet?	☐	☐
2. Any family history of polyps in the colon?	☐	☐
3. Any history of polyp removed from the colon?	☐	☐
4. Any history of treatment for ulcerative colitis?	☐	☐
5. Any history of alcohol use?	☐	☐

C. Health Habits

	YES	NO
1. Do you check your stool for hidden blood?	☐	☐

The more YES answers you have given to the above questions, the higher risk you have for that particular cancer.

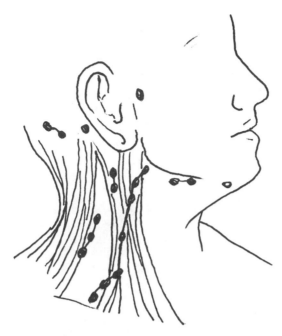

SELF EXAM: Lymph Nodes in the Neck
Reprinted with permission from Barbara Bates, M.D., *A Guide to Physical Examination*, B. Lippincott Co. 1974, pgs.45, 147, 217.

II. SELF EXAMINATIONS

Self examinations have proven to be very worthwhile in the early detection and prevention of cancer. For example, a large number of breast cancers are detected by the patients themselves. In considering the examples of breast cancer, the principle of early detection has been applied to other cancers and has been found to be quite effective.

The advantages of the self-exam is that it is cost effective, and large populations can use it at no expense after they have learned the technique. The disadvantages are that many people do not feel that self-exams are important, and many patients don't do a thorough job of examining themselves for cancer. For example, breast self-exams get poor marks because women do not do it often enough.

Lymph Nodes

Lymph nodes are part of the body's immune system. Many lymph nodes are located on both sides of the neck, in the armpits and in the

221

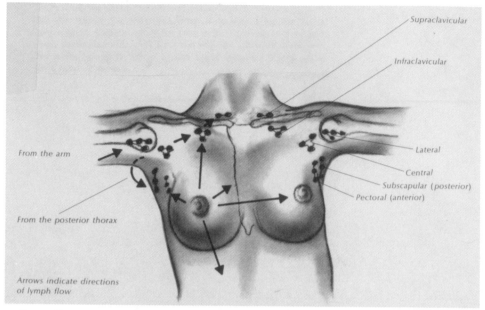

SELF EXAM: Lymph Nodes under Arms
Reprinted with permission from Barbara Bates, M.D., *A Guide to Physical Examination*, B. Lippincott Company, 1974, p. 45, 147, 217.

groin. People doing a self examination for the lymph nodes should visually examine the neck, armpit and the groin area in a brightly lit room (e.g., a bathroom), checking for any swelling. Next, by using the pads of the fingers, we can examine the neck, armpit or groin, rolling the fingers back and forth to feel for any swelling.

When examining the neck, it is important that the muscles be relaxed on the side being examined by tilting the head toward that side.

When the armpit is examined, the arm must be raised. With the other hand, reach as high into the armpit as possible, feeling for any swelling.

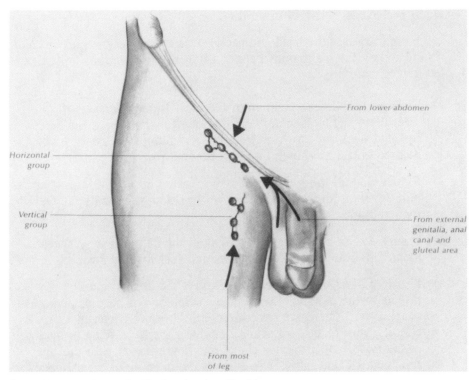

From lower abdomen

Horizontal group

Vertical group

From external genitalia, anal canal and gluteal area

From most of leg

SELF EXAM: Lymph Nodes in the Groin

Reprinted with permission from Barbara Bates, M.D., A Guide to Physical Examination, B. Lippincott Company, ©1974, p.45, 147, 217.

Check the glands in the groin by rolling the fingers at the top of the legs in the groin.

Head and Neck Self-Examination

Examination of the head and neck for cancer is very important. You should follow the eight steps below, using the illustrations on the next few pages, carefully.

1) **Figures 1 & 2.** Examination of the face. Remove glasses if you wear them and look in the mirror. Look for the skin of the face, lips and neck for any raised lumps and bumps or any scars or colored areas, as shown on the following page.

2) **Figure 3.** Pull the lower lip down to examine it first, and later pull upper lip upwards to look for any change in color or feel for any lumps or bumps.

3) **Figure 4.** Look at the gums. Take out the dentures if you wear them. Look for any color changes and feel for any swelling.

4) **Figure 5.** For the inner cheek. Expose the area by putting two fingers in the mouth. Look for any white or red patches or any rough spots. There are two things on the inner cheek that may concern you. One is the white line that runs from front to back in the middle of the inner cheek that corresponds with the bite and is called linea alba. The other is the opening of the salivary gland which is like a small red spot. Both of these things are normal.

5) **Figures 6 and 7.** Tongue and the floor of the mouth. Stick the tongue out and look at its top and edges as far as you can see. Then look at the floor of the mouth, by turning the tip of the tongue toward the roof of the mouth and look at the under-surface of the tongue. Feel with your finger for any lumps or bumps.

6) **Figure 8.** The roof of the mouth. Tilt your head back and look at the roof of the mouth by opening the mouth wide for any color changes, or lumps and bumps.

7) **Figure 9.** Examine the sides of the neck by running your fingers up and down, feeling for any lumps.

8) **Figure 10.** Examine the windpipe and thyroid gland. First feel the Adam's Apple then run your fingers down and feel for the thyroid gland. This gland is like a shield and sits in the front and sides of the lower part of the windpipe. Since it moves with swallowing, you can see it moving in the mirror.

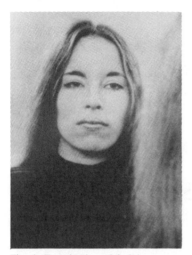

Fig. 1. Examination of facial symmetry.

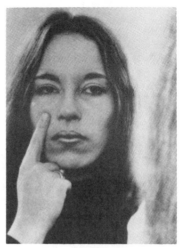

Fig. 2. Palpitation of the face.

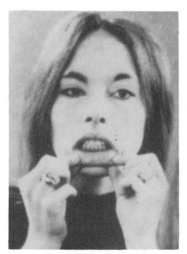

Fig. 3. Examination of lips.

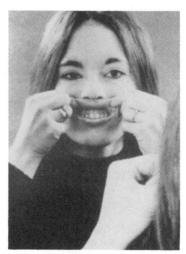

Fig. 4. Examination of gingiva.

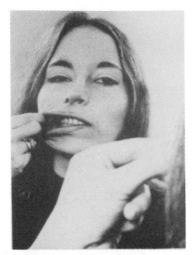

Fig. 5. Examination of buccal mucosa.

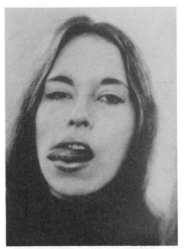

Fig. 6. Examination of tongue and floor of mouth.

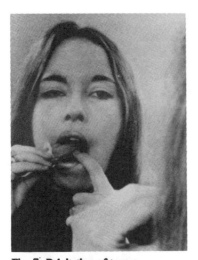

Fig. 7. Palpitation of tongue.

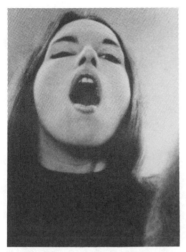

Fig. 8. Examination of palate.

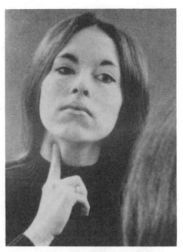

Fig. 9. Examination of lateral neck.

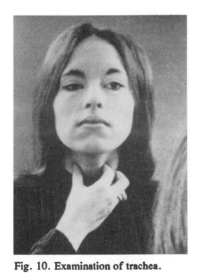

Fig. 10. Examination of trachea.

Self-Examination of Head and Neck, reprinted with permission by the American Dental Association.

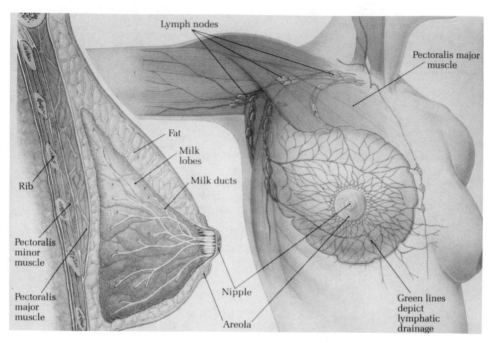

ANATOMY OF THE FEMALE BREAST *The breast is made up of ducts, lobes, lobules, fibrous tissue, and fat, with underlying muscle and bone (ribs). Therefore, it is normal for the breasts to feel lumpy or uneven. Before your menstrual period begins, and sometimes during your period, you can have some tenderness, pain, or lumps in your breasts because extra fluid collects in the tissue. This is normal.*

Breast Self-Examination

Breast Self Examination (BSE) is an inexpensive, non-invasive no-risk method of early breast cancer detection. Evidence and numerous studies say that breast cancer self-examination works.

A STEP-BY-STEP GUIDE TO BREAST SELF EXAMINATION [1]

A woman's breasts change throughout her life. Factors such as age, monthly menstrual cycle, pregnancy, breast feeding, birth control or

---

* Copies of the Breast Self-Examination Guide are available in full color. Patients may send $2. for each copy desired to: Breast Self-Examination Guide, Dominus Publishing Co., Inc., P.O. Box 86, Williston Park, NY 11596. Bulk prices also available. Be sure to include your name and address.

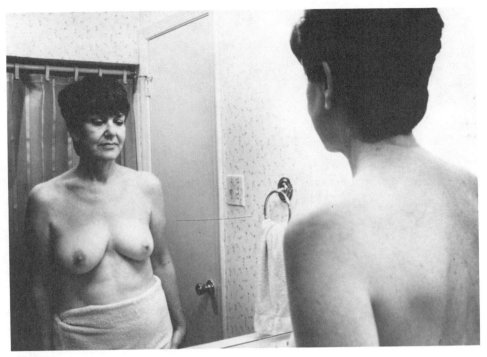

STEP 1

Stand before a mirror. Inspect both breasts for anything unusual, such as any discharge from the nipples, puckering, dimpling, or scaling of the skin. Each time you examine your breasts you will become more familiar with how they appear and feel, making it easier to notice any changes that may occur. Notice the normal size and shape of each breast (it is not unusual for one breast to be larger than the other) and the normal position of the nipple.

other hormone pills, menopause, or a bruise or blow to the breast can cause these changes. In addition, breasts vary in size, shape and texture. Because over 70 percent of all breast lumps are found by women themselves, you should learn how to examine your breasts monthly. As you do this, you will develop more confidence in knowing how your breasts normally feel and should be able to recognize any changes. If you do find a change, don't let fear keep you from seeing your doctor. When breast cancer is found early, the chances are better for survival and for less disfiguring treatment. In fact, there are now many more options than radical surgery.

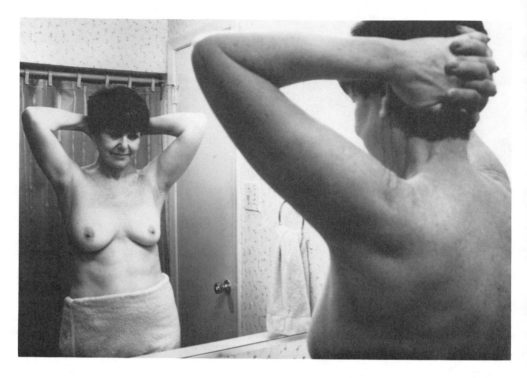

STEP 2

Clasp your hands behind your head and press them forward. Look in the mirror at the shape and contour of your breasts. Take your time; again look for any changes in the size and shape of each breast and look for any swelling, dimpling, rash, discoloration, or other unusual changes of the skin.

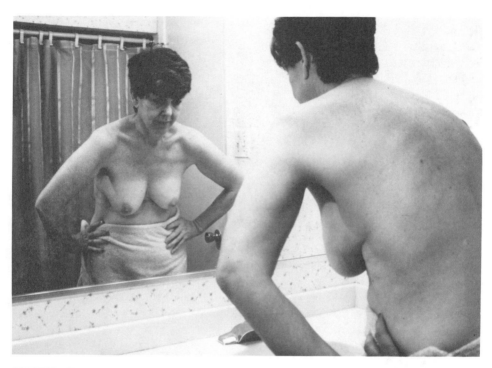

STEP 3

Next, press your hands firmly on your hips and bow slightly toward your mirror as you pull your shoulders and elbows forward. Once again, look for any change in the shape or contour of your breasts.

Some women do the next part of the exam in the shower. Fingers glide over soapy skin, making it easy to concentrate on the texture underneath. Raise your left arm. Use three or four fingers of your right hand to explore your left breast firmly, carefully, and thoroughly. Keep your fingers flat and close together. Use enough pressure to feel deep into the breast, but not so much to dull your sensations. With practice, you'll learn how much pressure to use.

231

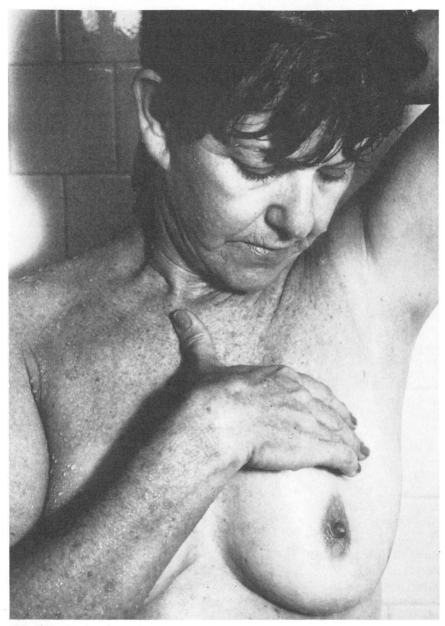

STEP 4
Beginning at the outer edge, press the flat part of your fingers in small
circles, moving the circles slowly around the breast. Gradually work

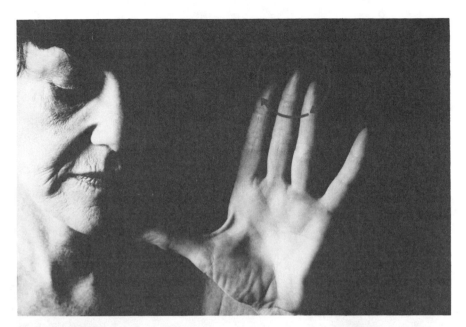

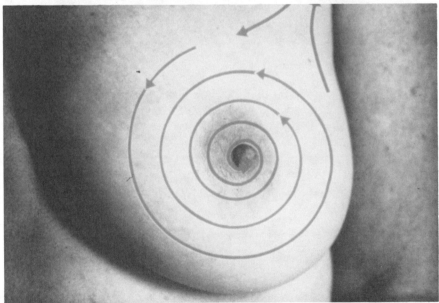

toward the nipple. Be sure to cover the entire breast. Pay special attention to the area between the breast and the armpit, including the armpit itself. Feel for any unusual lump or mass under the skin. A lump is unusual if it has not been felt during earlier breast exams and it now stands out against the normal feel of your breast.

233

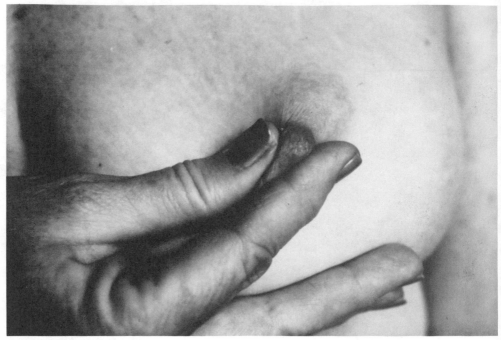

STEP 5

Gently squeeze the nipple and look for a discharge. If present, see your doctor. In fact, if you have a discharge at any time you should check it out with your doctor. Repeat steps 4 and 5 on your right breast.

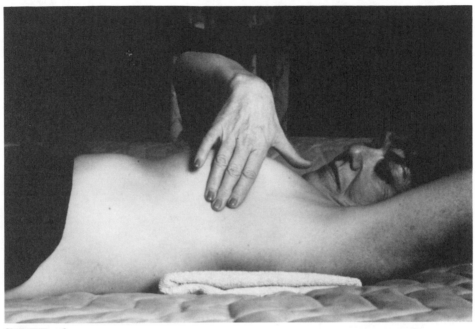

STEP 6

Repeat steps 4 and 5 lying down. Lie flat on your back, left arm over your head and a pillow or folded towel under your left shoulder. This position flattens the breast and makes it easier to examine. Use the same circular motion described earlier. Repeat on your right breast. If your breasts are large, you may need to hold the side of each one steady, either with your other hand or by resting it against a wall.

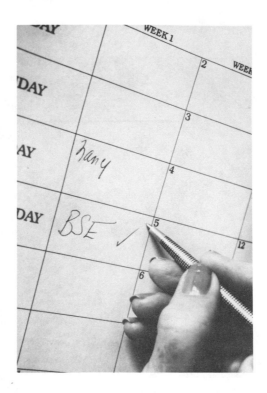

STEP 7

If you feel something in one breast that appears unusual or different from before, check to see if it is present in your other breast. If the same structure is in the same place in both breasts, the chances are good that your breasts are normal. If you find a lump a few days before or during your menstrual period, reexamine your breasts when your period ends. Often a lump found at this time may be due to the normal collection of fluid during your period. If the lump doesn't disappear before your next period begins, see your doctor soon.

Breast self examination should be done once a month. If you menstruate, the best time to do BSE is two or three days after your period ends, when your breasts are least likely to be tender or swollen. If you no longer menstruate, pick a day, such as the first day of the month, to remind yourself it is time to do BSE and write it down. If you are just learning how to examine your breasts, you may want to do BSE once a week for a couple of months to see how your breasts change over time. Once you know what is normal for you, then just do it once a month.

Look out below

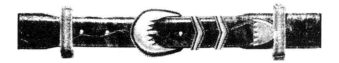

It's time you gave yourself a GSE™

©BURROUGHS WELLCOME CO.

GENITAL SELF EXAM CAMPAIGN
Reprinted with permission from Jerry Breitman, *American Medical News,* August 1989.

Genital Self-Examination

FOR WOMEN: VULVAR SELF-EXAMINATION

Women should perform vulvar self-examination for any itching, growth, lump or sore or an ulcer. The inspection should be done in good light and with a hand-mirror. You can stand with one foot on a stool. The outer vulva should be inspected all the way down to the anus. Continue the inspection on the outer and inner lips, clitoris and vagina and inner labia. Then the skin should be palpated for any swelling that could not be seen. Caution should be exercised that no talcum powder is used in the examined area.

FOR MEN: TESTICULAR AND PENILE SELF-EXAMINATION

For men and young boys there are two parts to examination. The first is to examine the testicles and the other is for the penis.

Since testicle cancer is the most common cancer in 15 to 34-year-old men, the best way to teach this age group is at the high school and middle school level. In a letter published in the *New England Journal of Medicine*, Drs. Garnick, Mayer, and Richie of Dana Farber Cancer Institute wrote about a very interesting story. A film projectionist, a 29-year-old man employed at the institute, viewed the film on testicular self-examination on two separate occasions. It was reported that he

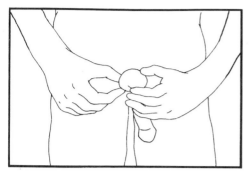 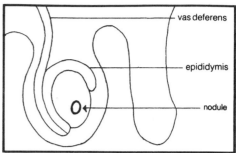

FOR MEN ONLY: TESTICULAR CANCER AND HOW TO DO TSE (A Self Exam), Reprinted with permission from the American Cancer Society, Inc., ©American Cancer Socity, Pamphlet #82-250M, No. 2093 - LE

examined his own testicle and found a bean sized lump in the right testicle.

First, you should inspect the testicles in good light to see if there is any asymmetry (difference in size or shape). Second, you can palpate them by holding the testicle between thumb and index finger of both hands, one at a time, and roll the testicles between the finger and the thumb and feel for any lesion shaped like a pea or a bean. It's best to do the examination in a warm shower when the scrotal skin is warm and relaxed.

Parents of young boys should also be taught to examine the testicles of their children.

Because genital warts are pre-cancerous lesions, it is important that regular penile self-examination is done on a monthly basis. It should be done in good light and preferably in a warm room. Look for any warts, redness, and persistent itchy or flaky areas. The skin should be palpated by hand for any lumps and the groin should be checked for any enlarged lymph nodes.

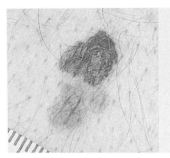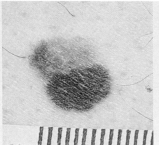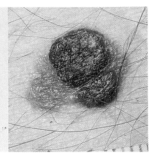

LEFT: Level III tumor, 1.2 mm thick.
CENTER: Level II tumor, 0.3 mm thick.
RIGHT: Level II tumor, 0.6 mm thick.

Melanomas are disorderly in appearance, with irregular and/or discontinuous pigmentation (brown, black, blue-black, gray and pink), irregular borders, and irregular surface elevation or nodularity. Melanomas developed contiguous with dysplastic moles. Rules are in millimeters.[2]

Skin Self-Examination

Skin self examination is very important for people of all ages. If you have any moles or lesions, they should be mapped and measured or checked on a monthly basis. You should have an annual skin exam done by your physician.

The full body diagrams on the following pages illustrate in ten simple steps a method of conducting a full body skin self-examination.

You should look for moles which are the size of this circle ◯ (six millimeters in diameter) or larger, have varied color mixtures of tan, brown, black or red/pink, and have irregular borders with a flat portion level with the skin, often at the edge of the mole. Pay special attention to areas which get exposed to the sun.

The typical adult has ten to 40 moles scattered over the body. If you have significantly more than 40 moles, you should conduct this self-exam routinely.

*Reproduced with permission from "Cutaneous Melanoma," Arthur R. Rhodes, M.D., *Journal of the American Medical Association*, Pgs. 3148/3149 Vol. 258, No.21, Dec. 4, 1987, ©1987, American Medical Association.

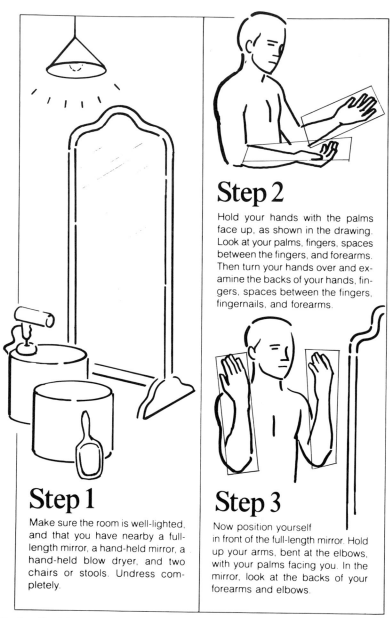

Step 2

Hold your hands with the palms face up, as shown in the drawing. Look at your palms, fingers, spaces between the fingers, and forearms. Then turn your hands over and examine the backs of your hands, fingers, spaces between the fingers, fingernails, and forearms.

Step 1

Make sure the room is well-lighted, and that you have nearby a full-length mirror, a hand-held mirror, a hand-held blow dryer, and two chairs or stools. Undress completely.

Step 3

Now position yourself in front of the full-length mirror. Hold up your arms, bent at the elbows, with your palms facing you. In the mirror, look at the backs of your forearms and elbows.

Body Self Exam

Reprinted with permission from *CA-A Cancer Journal for Clinicians*, Vol. 35, No.3 May/June 1985.

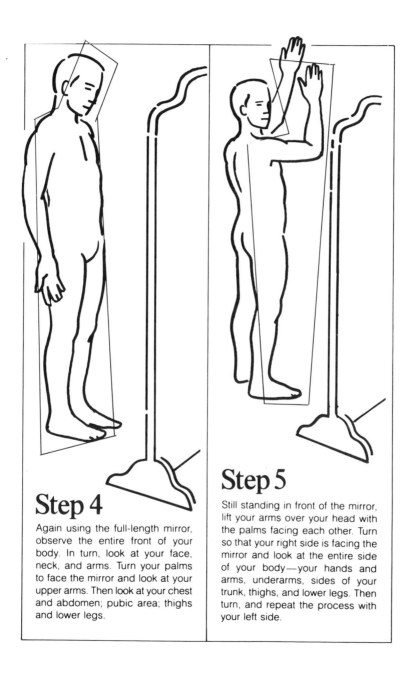

Step 4

Again using the full-length mirror, observe the entire front of your body. In turn, look at your face, neck, and arms. Turn your palms to face the mirror and look at your upper arms. Then look at your chest and abdomen; pubic area; thighs and lower legs.

Step 5

Still standing in front of the mirror, lift your arms over your head with the palms facing each other. Turn so that your right side is facing the mirror and look at the entire side of your body—your hands and arms, underarms, sides of your trunk, thighs, and lower legs. Then turn, and repeat the process with your left side.

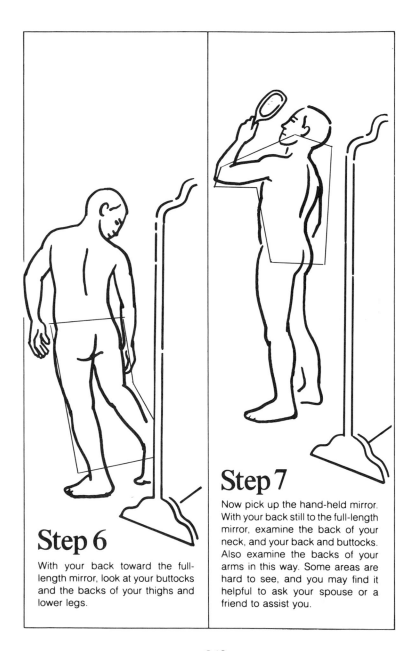

Step 6

With your back toward the full-length mirror, look at your buttocks and the backs of your thighs and lower legs.

Step 7

Now pick up the hand-held mirror. With your back still to the full-length mirror, examine the back of your neck, and your back and buttocks. Also examine the backs of your arms in this way. Some areas are hard to see, and you may find it helpful to ask your spouse or a friend to assist you.

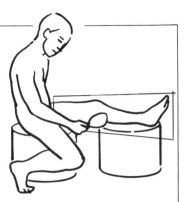

Step 9

Sit down and prop up one leg on a chair or stool in front of you as shown. Using the hand-held mirror, examine the inside of the propped-up leg, beginning at the groin area and moving the mirror down the leg to your foot. Repeat the procedure for your other leg.

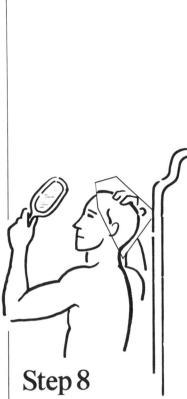

Step 8

Use the hand-held mirror and the full-length mirror to look at your scalp. Because the scalp is difficult to examine, we suggest you also use a hand-held blow dryer turned to a cool setting, to lift the hair from the scalp. While some people find it easy to hold the mirror in one hand and the dryer in the other, while looking in the full-length mirror, many do not. For the scalp examination in particular, then, you might ask your spouse or a friend to assist you.

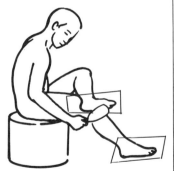

Step 10

Still sitting, cross one leg over the other. Use the hand-held mirror to examine the top of your foot, the toes, toenails, and spaces between the toes. Then look at the sole or bottom of your foot. Repeat the procedure for the other foot.

243

III. SCREENING PROGRAMS

Screening programs for the following cancers have been designed with the premise that early detection will lead to early diagnosis and eventually lowered mortality rates and more cures in cancer.

In today's cost-conscious society, it is very important that we use our resources very carefully. If we decide to examine large segments of the population for certain cancers, it is very important that we design cost-conscious screening programs.

The first screening programs were:

1. PAP SMEARS FOR CERVICAL CANCER. The American Cancer Society started education of the public using the slogan, "let no woman be overlooked." The use of Pap smears have already yielded great results and lowered mortality rates. The test has been very widely used and accepted.
2. BREAST CANCER. The HIP 1962 study by a New York Insurance Company showed early detection of breast cancer led to lower mortality rates. Through breast exams and mammographies, many cancers have been detected in early stages.
3. COLORECTAL CANCER. In the past few years, the American Cancer Society has launched a great campaign to educate the public. The occult blood test is designed for those over 40. Sigmoidoscopy follows a rectal exam.
4. ENDOMETRIAL CANCER. Patients at a high risk of cancer of the mucous lining of the uterus often have endometrial tests for cytology.
5. PROSTATE CANCER. The rectal exam is the best screening test. Suspicious areas can be confirmed with ultrasound against the prostate.
6. SKIN CANCER. Since malignant melanoma rates are very high in Australia, The Australian Cancer Society has taken the lead in educating the public about the dangers of solar radiation. The group has designed screening programs for the general public at health fairs and has been very successful.
7. ORAL CANCER. This can be done during dental exam or at health fairs. Oral cancer is very easy to detect and these screening programs are especially appropriate for the southern United States, where many chew tobacco.
8. THYROID CANCER. The Michael Reese Hospital in Chicago has a program of follow-up of patients who were given radiation to the head and neck for benign conditions. The Life Span Study in Hiroshima and Nagasaki of radiation exposure victims also

indicates the importance of screening for thyroid cancer. Now, the victims of the Chernobyl nuclear accident, nearly 100,000 people, will be followed.

9. TESTICULAR CANCER. This screening is appropriate for the 15-35 year age group. The program can be easily designed in schools for early detection for testicular cancer and can be incorporated with a movie about self exams.

10. ESOPHAGEAL CANCER. The highest rates of esophageal cancer are in China, especially in the Hunan province. The "balloon test" is designed for early detection, similar to use of the Pap test. A balloon-like instrument is inserted down the esophagus. If cancer cells are present some will shed and attach to the balloon. The material on the balloon is then tested for cancerous cells. This is quite an effective screening program.

11. STOMACH CANCER. The highest rates of stomach cancer are in Japan. Endoscopy is often used for screening.

12. LIVER CANCER. The blood test Serial AFP monitoring studies in Eskimos in Alaska have been found to be very successful in hepatic cancer.

13. BLADDER CANCER. Smoking and occupational exposures must be stopped or at least decreased to cut down on this cancer.

Examination by Physician

Screening for cancer can also be done in the physician's office even on a routine visit. The role of the annual physical exam is very important. During each visit, the patient should be educated about preventive practices such as quitting smoking, reducing alcohol intake, and monitoring living and working environment. The skin, oral cavity, thyroid, lymph nodes, etc., can be checked and self-examination techniques taught to the patient. Weight loss and any other symptoms suggesting cancer should be followed up.

The office nurse can serve as a good reminder to patients of physical exams. In offices where nurses reminded patients to maintain their health by getting periodic health examinations, there is a significant increase in performance of the following examinations:

1. Pap smear;
2. Fecal occult blood exam; and
3. Breast examination.

The following schedule has been adapted from the American Cancer Society guidelines.

Summary of American Cancer Society Recommendations for the Early Detection of Cancer in Asymptomatic People

Test or Procedure		Sex	Age	Frequency
Colon:	Sigmoidoscopy	M & F	Over 50	Every 3-5 years.
	Stool Guaiac Slide Test	M & F	Over 50	Every year.
	Digital Rectal	M & F	Over 40	Every year.
Cervix:	Pap Test	F	18-65; Under 18, if sexually active.	Annually until 3 consecutive normal exams, then at physicians discretion.
Ovarian:	Pelvic Examination	F	20-40 Over 40.	Every 3 years. Every year.
Endo:	Endometrial Tissue Sample	F	At menopause, if at high risk.*	
Breast:	Breast Self Examination	F	Over 20	Every month
	Breast Physical Examination	F	20-40 Over 40	Every 3 years. Every year.
	Mammography	F	Between 35-39 40-49 Over 50	Baseline Every 1-2 years. Every year.
Lung:	Chest X-ray			Not recommended.
	Sputum Cytology			Not recommended.
	Health Counseling and Cancer Check-Up**	M & F	Over 20 Over 40	Every 3 years. Every year.

* History of infertility, obesity, failure to ovulate, abnormal uterine bleeding, or estrogen therapy.
** To include examination for cancers of the thyroid, testicles, prostate, ovaries, lymph nodes, oral region, and skin.

American Cancer Society, Dec. 1989. *Ca — A Cancer Journal for Clinicians*, 1990: 40(2):79

CONCLUSION

NEW FRONTIERS IN CANCER PREVENTION

Western society will face tremendous changes in the coming years. One of the most significant is that by the year 2050, one-third of the United States' population will be fifty-five or older.[1] Generally, cancer is a disease affecting the older age group; its incidence is also rising at the rate of one percent yearly, making it a substantial challenge for scientists. Another significant change will be that fewer young people will be supporting this burgeoning older population. As a result, the economy will play a major role in how we handle the problems incurred by an aging population, including those of cancer prevention and treatment. Since treatment of cancer is expensive, progress made on longevity with surgery, radiation and chemotherapy will be comparatively small. Instead, prevention techniques will be pushed to the forefront of all medicine, cancer not excepted, by future changes in demographics and economics, as well as the rapid pace of technological advances. It is becoming more important than ever that infants are given a healthy start, enabling them to reduce the chronic sickness caused by environmental conditions and by personal lifestyles. Also of increased importance is maintaining the health and independence of the elderly.[2]

Will we be able to cure cancer in our lifetime? This question was dealt with by a number of scientists at the Prevention 89 convention in

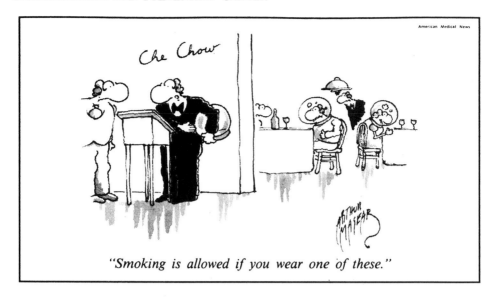

"Smoking is allowed if you wear one of these."

Reprinted with permission from *American Medical News*, and Scott Arthur Masear.

Atlanta. The answer was "maybe." Dr. Richard Streckel, Director of Jonsson Comprehensive Cancer Center at the University of California, feels that there will be a breakthrough in cancer prevention stemming from the advances in molecular biology. Sixty-three percent of the researchers polled felt better prevention will do more than treatment or diagnosis to fight cancer by the year 2000.[3]

CAUSES OF CANCER AND SOLUTIONS

Tobacco and Marijuana

Tobacco and marijuana continue to be the most avoidable causes of cancer. We are all familiar with the worldwide economic and political power of tobacco interests, so we realize that it is not going to disappear overnight. But the tobacco industry is losing ground in the legal debate over smoking in public areas because of the dangers of second-hand smoke. When smoking becomes socially unacceptable, the nails will have been hammered into the coffin of the tobacco industry. Once the words "death" and "addiction" are added to the surgeon general's warning on cigarette cartons, I predict that there will be a spate of lawsuits against tobacco companies. Tobacco industry representatives will have to sit next to asbestos company representatives in the courtrooms for causing cancer deaths. Sadly, chewing tobacco—as addicting and cancer-causing as cigarette smoke—is making a comeback; baseball stars could help curb this trend by not promoting it. Finally, marijuana, which contains carcinogenic chemicals, should be seen as a recreational drug which is deadly.

Sunlight

The continued production and use of chlorofluorocarbons means that there will be further depletion of the ozone layer—leading to an increase in the amount of dangerous ultraviolet B radiation from the sun that reaches the earth. The number of skin cancers in general, and of melanoma in particular, will increase accordingly. It is estimated that there will be approximately 31,000 to 126,000 cases of melanoma in the United States in whites born before 2075, resulting in 7,000-30,000 deaths.[4]

Exposure to ultraviolet light not only causes skin cancer, but also suppresses the immune system. I believe this explains the increased number of pneumonias in my own patients at the start of the summer when everyone goes out into the sun.

In addition to taking measures to protect the ozone, we need to impose some sort of restrictions on the tanning facilities which have become so popular among the health and exercise clubs in our appearance-conscious America.

Ionizing Radiation

Atomic power, one source of ionizing radiation, is on its way out. Nuclear power plants turned out to be white elephants: they were not as cost-effective as had been publicized initially. New York citizens were able to shut down the Shoreham Nuclear Power Plant before it even began operating. We still need to develop better ways to store existing radioactive waste, and to curtail the waste still being produced.

Diagnostic X-rays will continue to be improved, using lower doses of radiation and faster film, so that the risk to patients will be minimal. Changes in malpractice laws will hopefully curtail unnecessary use of X-rays.

Finally, natural sources of radiation need to be measured and curtailed. We will see more regulation in construction codes in houses and buildings to reduce entry of radon. Also, pregnant airline crew members will be restricted from high altitude flying, so that the fetus is not exposed to cosmic radiation.

Chemicals

We seem to have a "chemical solution" to every household problem, a spray for every bug or weed. We need to change our way of thinking and use less-harmful substances to solve our cleaning needs. Asbestos is everywhere, in schools, houses, office buildings, and getting into our lungs. It is best to encapsulate asbestos and remove it carefully if the building has to be renovated. Further manufacture of asbestos should be banned completely. Benzene and other solvents are still around, but we must find and use less dangerous substitutes.

Plastics and pesticides are a primary cause for the destruction of the environment. Of all chemicals, pesticides deserve the highest dishonorable mention. Farmers need to be educated in integrated pest management, and weed killers should be banned for use in backyard lawns. Pesticide companies should not use the word "treat" for something that stands for pesticide poisoning of the environment.

Finally, it is critical that we develop a "cradle to grave" philosophy for the use of all chemicals; there must be proper accounting for these dangerous chemicals from creation to destruction. Hazardous waste should be handled by a new plan called Integrated Waste Management, with a focus on recycling.

Diet

Diet will play a key role in future control and prevention of cancer, with an emphasis on low-fat and high fiber content. Most effective in the use of diet to fight cancer are vitamins and minerals. A powerful tool in the battle against cancer are the vitamin A derivatives called Retinoids—applied topically and administered orally—and already proven to be effective in the chemoprevention trials under the auspices of the National Cancer Institute.

According to *Prevention Magazine*, a larger segment of the population in the 21st century will be vegetarian. Organically grown vegetables and fruits will become increasingly popular, and supermarkets will promise to carry only pesticide-free produce. People will eat more fish from fish farms. Genetically engineered beta carotene-rich honeydew melons, cantaloupes and watermelons will be plentiful.

We know from many recent reports about the efficacy of fiber in reducing the incidence of colon cancer in patients with polyps of the colon and in preventing a recurrence in patients who have already had colon cancer. As more and more of the population switches to a high fiber and low-fat diet, low in cholesterol, we should see a significant reduction in the incidence of colon cancer.

Contagious Cancers and the Immune System

For cancers caused by infectious agents, the role of the immune system will become of utmost importance. People will learn how to reduce damage to their immune system by avoiding tobacco, radiation chemicals, and dietary factors that interfere with proper functioning of the immune system or which deplete it. They will also learn how to boost their immune system with dietary manipulation, psychology and exercise.

Since the immune system will no longer be such a mystery, scientists will design ways in which the different components can be controlled and stimulated to our advantage. In a group of scientists polled recently, 88 percent felt that drugs that stimulate the immune system will play an important role in the future.[5] As we already know, we can boost the immune system with a BCG vaccine, and interferons and interleukins have been an important discovery. The vaccines against some cancer-causing viruses are already here, such as those for hepatitis-B and feline leukemia. We desperately need a vaccine for AIDS and human papilloma viruses.

Finally, the era of cancer vaccines is here. They are already being used against a number of cancers, and 86 percent of the research scientists in this country believe that development of genetically engineered vaccines is the most promising area of applied research, while the resulting vaccines will have the highest impact on modern medicine.[6]

Hormones and Chemotherapy

The use of hormones will continue declining and doses will become smaller—something we have already seen in the case of birth control pills and post-menopausal estrogens. Steroids will probably become illegal in the near future.

The use of chemotherapy and radiation to control cancer will subside as vitamin derivatives and immune system boosters take over the field of cancer treatment. The combined effect of different treatments will be less than the benefits accrued from preventative measures, says Dr. Saul Rosenberg, Chief of Oncology at Stanford University. Quitting smoking can have more impact on cancer than all other treatments combined.[7]

Hereditary Cancers

The major breakthrough in hereditary cancers is likely to come from molecular biology research, enabling us to repair hereditary damage to genes. Improved tests for the cancer-prone will be developed, and there will be better follow-up for cancer families. Genetic research is moving at a fast pace, allowing prevention to move to the root of the problem in cancer.[8] The Nobel Prize for Medicine in 1989 went to Drs. Michael Bishop and Howard Varmus of the University of California, who were rewarded for their oncogene research in the late 1970s.

Pollution

Pollution knows no boundaries. Soil may be the property of a particular country, but air and water are not. Any pollution of air and water will end up in the soil, from where it will move to the food chain and on to the ultimate victim, human beings. Protection of the environment has to be a global effort. Governments cannot act as guardians of every square inch of land, so it is our responsibility, as good citizens and for the sake of our children, to safeguard the environment. We have only one earth on which to live.

We can still take many steps to protect the environment, but time is running out. Environmental pollution should be a top priority of all governments, schools, and public education programs. Fortunately, a number of grass roots movements have already started the process.

CONCLUSION NOTES

1. *Medical Tribune*, (Jan. 14, 1988)
2. J. Michael McGinnis, Office of Disease Prevention and Health Promotion, Prevention '89 Convention, Atlanta, Georgia.
3. Richard Streckel, *Medical Tribune*, (Jan. 1988)
4. Worldwatch Institute Report, *New England Journal of Medicine*, (Dec. 7, 1989)
5. *Medical Tribune*, Prevention 89 Convention
6. Saul Rosenberg, *Medical Tribune*, (Jan. 1988)
7. *Ibid.*
8. Beverly Merz, *Journal of the American Medical Association*, (Nov. 24, 1989)

I trust this effort, A FAMILY DOCTOR'S GUIDE TO UNDERSTANDING AND PREVENTING CANCER, will lead to improved understanding of the causes of cancer and the various protective health measures we, as individuals, can take to reduce our risk of the dreaded disease.

As with any public health measure, to be effective a message has to reach the right people at the right time.[1] The right people are everyone: children, adults and the elderly, in this country and in the rest of the world. The right time is now, because these people have not yet developed cancer.

It is my sincere hope that reading this book and acting on the advice given will not only improve the quality of life for all of us, but also protect our environment and save lives around the world. If even one person benefits, I will consider my eight years of hard work on this book — a mission accomplished.

S.R. Kaura, M.D.

---

[1] Jerome Marmorstein, *Medical Tribune.*

GLOSSARY

ADENOMA: A benign tumor of glandular tissue. It can be precancerous in cases such as polyps in the colon.

AFLATOXINS: Poisonous compounds produced by a fungus in moldy foods.

ANTIBODY: A protein manufactured by cells of the immune system to counteract antigens.

ANTIGENS: Foreign materials like bacteria, viruses and toxins, which create a slow allergic reaction over 8 to 14 days. The body reacts by making antibodies.

AROMATIC AMINES: Petrochemical compounds with pungent odor known to cause cancer in human beings.

BARIUM ENEMA: A test in which barium is used as a contrast to do X-rays of the colon. It is used as a test for cancer.

BCG: A vaccine to prevent tuberculosis. Also used to stimulate the immune system against cancer.

BENIGN TUMOR: An abnormal collection of healthy looking cells that are slow growing (faster than normal cells, slower than cancer cells). These tumors do not spread into other areas of the body, unlike cancerous tumors. They do their damage by putting pressure on normally healthy areas. Some benign tumors can become malignant.

BIOMAGNIFICATION: The name given to a process in which small bugs contaminated with toxic chemicals are eaten by larger bugs, the larger bugs by animals, and then the animals by human beings, with each step concentrating the poison thousands of times.

BURKITT'S LYMPHOMA: A tumor of the lymphatic tissues of the neck and face, commonly seen in African children.

CARCINOGENESIS: A biological process changing the normal cell into a cancer cell.

CARCINOGENS: Agents that can cause cancer.

CARCINOMA: A malignant tumor of the cells lining the gut, lung, airways and skin, starting in epithelial tissues. Representing 85-90 percent of all cancers.

CO-CARCINOGENS: Agents that assist carcinogens in causing cancer.

COLONOSCOPY: A test in which a flexible tube with a light is inserted into the rectum to view the inside of the colon.

COMPLETE CARCINOGENS: agents that will both initiate and promote.

CULDOSCOPY: A magnified examination of the cervix for precancerous stages.

DYSPLASTIC NEVI SYNDROME: Abnormal moles that can change into a melanoma, often occurring in many members of the same family.

GAMMA RAYS: Extremely short electromagnetic waves that are transmitted by nuclear material like radium and Cobalt 60.

IMMUNOTHERAPY: A way to boost the immune system as a whole or strengthen different components of the immune system to fight infections or cancer.

INITIATORS: Agents that cause permanent damage to the DNA.

INTERLEUKIN 2 AND INTERFERON: These are compounds produced by the immune system to fight infections or cancer. They are available as medications.

LARYNGEAL CANCER: Cancer of the voice box.

LEUKEMIA: An abnormal number of white cells produced in the bone marrow, representing four percent of all cancers.

LEUKOPLAKIA: White patches in the mouth which become cancerous in approximately three percent of patients.

LYMPHOMA: A cancer starting from white cells of the lymph nodes, spleen, central nervous system, and bowel, representing about five percent of all cancers.

LYMPHOMAS: Malignant tumors of the lymphatic tissue.

MALIGNANT TUMOR: Cancer which has spread into neighboring tissues and distant organs.

MELANOMA: Cancers of the pigment cells or melanocytes of the skin or eyes.

MIXED: Mixture of carcinoma and sarcoma.

MULTIPLE MYELOMA: A cancer starting in plasma cells of bone marrow.

MUTAGENS: Agents that can cause initiation or mutations when tested on laboratory bacteria.

NASOPHARYNGEAL CARCINOMA: Cancer of the throat commonly seen in Asian countries because of Epstein-Barr Virus.

NON-HODGKIN'S LYMPHOMAS: Cancer of the lymphatic tissue.

OSTEOGENIC SARCOMA: Bone cancer.

PHOTOCARCINOGENESIS: Study of the carcinogenic effects of ultraviolet light.

POLYPS: Benign tumors in the colon or larynx.

PRO-CARCINOGENS: Agents that are not carcinogenic by themselves but are metabolized by the body into carcinogens.

PROMOTERS: Agents that only promote, acting on initiated cells.

RADIOISOTOPES: Nuclear materials used in medical diagnosis and treatment of medical conditions and in the pharmaceutical industry.

SARCOMA: Fleshy tumors of connective tissues, bones, muscle, fat cells, etc.

SPONTANEOUS REMISSION: A process by which the immune system causes the cancer to regress.

SPF: Sun Protection Factor or the degree of sun protection offered by a sunscreen. The higher the number of the sunblock, the greater the protection.

ULCERATIVE COLITIS: An inflammatory condition of the colon. If extensive and prolonged, it can lead to cancer of the colon.

WILM'S TUMOR: A cancer of the kidney in infants and children.

INDEX

259